Praise for *Periodic Bitch*

'Revelatory. Emma Hardy blends astute research and the poetry of pain in a word-perfect memoir. Clever, funny and assured, *Periodic Bitch* is essential reading that illuminates one of our least understood and most destructive illnesses. Through her candid and moving self-reflection, Hardy resolutely captures the heartache of having a uterus that's trying to kill you (and everyone else).' **Anna Spargo-Ryan, author of *A Kind of Magic***

'A beautiful literary memoir that is part detective story, part love story: why is the author like this? Can she love and be loved anyway? How do we make a life with someone, how do we work, write and create, when we can't even trust our own feelings? For those with PMDD, *Periodic Bitch* will be transformative—but all readers will gasp and admire how Emma Hardy captures the moment-by-moment experience of being alive.' **Jessica Stanley, author of *Consider Yourself Kissed***

'*Periodic Bitch* is much more than a medical memoir, it is an unflinching exploration of what it means to be human. Are we fleshy bags of hormones, Frankenstein monsters or social constructs; or are we, like the book, so wonderfully complex that we defy easy categorisation? Emma Hardy takes us to the dark places we didn't think we wanted to visit but she does so with such eloquence, intelligence and honesty that we are grateful for the experience.' **Melanie Cheng, author of *The Burrow***

'Hardy's memoir is ecological and medical, careful self-surgery and rigorous cultural dissection. She holds the thin shell that separates myth from our bodies, gendered bias from science, love from pain as it dissolves and reforms in her hands again and again. *Periodic Bitch* tracks the grinding cycles of everyday misogyny, existential uncertainty and the (sometimes) special powers of monstrosity in the same way it tracks the moods of Hardy's menstruation: you know it's coming, but how much damage might it cause? This work of menstrual poetics is intense and feral, as it must be.' **Hayley Singer, author of *Abandon Every Hope***

'*Periodic Bitch* is an expansive work of memoir, drawing on cinema, history and mythology as various lenses through which her own illness might be understood. Hardy is a frank and incisive narrator whose scrutiny exempts no one, least of all herself. By turns thought-provoking, rage-inducing and darkly funny, *Periodic Bitch* is a candid exploration of medical misogyny and the terror of the unknown: the strangeness of what it is to live with a poorly understood chronic condition.' **Jennifer Down, author of *Bodies of Light***

'From the bloodshot eye of a cyclone, Hardy gently points at each ring of PMDD's vortex with unmatched wit and curiosity, inviting her readers into the inner workings of its torrents.' **Madison Griffiths, author of *Sweet Nothings***

'*Periodic Bitch* offers a fiercely human corrective to the historically clinical explorations of menstrual and mental health with a unique magnetism. Author Emma Hardy brings an expansiveness to a shared time of lockdown, weaving her own journey and locality with stories from the worlds of art and medicine to expose the messiness of life and what it is to want to be able to truly live in the moment.' **Kate Jinx, writer and film curator**

Emma Hardy is an Australian writer based in Naarm/Melbourne. Her writing has been published in *Guernica*, *The Monthly*, *Los Angeles Review of Books*, *The Lifted Brow*, *Voiceworks* and *Going Down Swinging*. Emma lives with premenstrual dysphoric disorder, which is the topic of her debut book, *Periodic Bitch*. She often writes about women, animals, madness and the lines between. She has recently returned from three years living and writing in Nevada, where she was an MFA candidate at the University of Nevada, Las Vegas. She taught university-level English and creative writing and was the non-fiction editor at *Witness Magazine*.

PERIODIC BITCH

A memoir of menstruation, madness & monsters

EMMA HARDY

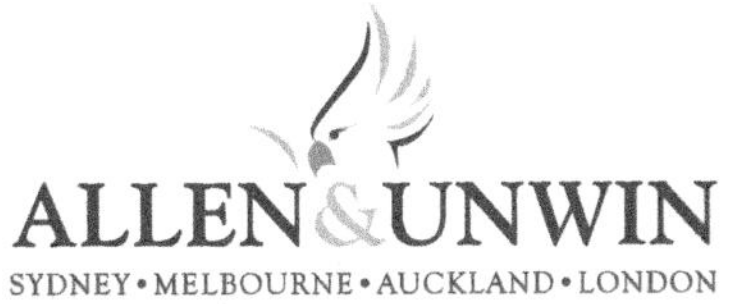

The information contained within this book is not intended to replace medical advice or to be relied upon to treat, cure or prevent any disease, illness or medical condition. The author and publisher claim no responsibility to any person or entity for any liability, loss or damage caused or alleged to be caused directly or indirectly as a result of the use, application or interpretation of the material in this book.

Content warning: This book describes an experience of menstrual illness known as premenstrual dysphoric disorder. It deals with themes that some readers may find uncomfortable or upsetting, including suicidal ideation, self-harm, disordered eating and drug use. It also explores themes of domestic violence, abortion, institutionalisation, ableism and medical sexism. Readers who are sensitive to these topics are advised discretion.

First published in 2026

Allen & Unwin
Cammeraygal Country
83 Alexander Street
Crows Nest NSW 2065
Australia
Phone: (61 2) 8425 0100
Email: info@allenandunwin.com
Web: www.allenandunwin.com

Allen & Unwin acknowledges the Traditional Owners of the Country on which we live and work. We pay our respects to all Aboriginal and Torres Strait Islander Elders, past and present.

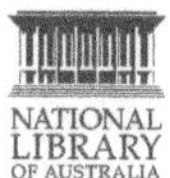

A catalogue record for this book is available from the National Library of Australia

ISBN 978 1 76147 359 3

Cover design: Hazel Lam
Cover images: Zhixin Li / Stocksy United; Wolf from Die Säugthiere in Abbildungen nach der Natur (1778–1855) by Georg August Goldfuss, Johann Andreas Wagener and Johann Christian Daniel von Schreber / rawpixel
Internal design: Bookhouse, Sydney
Set in 11.5/18 pt Bembo MT Pro by Bookhouse, Sydney
Printed and bound in Australia by the Opus Group

10 9 8 7 6 5 4 3 2

The paper in this book is FSC® certified. FSC® promotes environmentally responsible, socially beneficial and economically viable management of the world's forests.

To Pavan.
For better, for worse.

Prologue

Somewhere in the middle, Pavan snaps.

'No one else would be able to love you,' he says. 'No one else would put up with this.'

At first I am winded, shocked. Then I am relieved. His patience has finally given way. He has said the most horrible thing. Finally, I have something real to be upset about.

I cross the road to get away from him, start cry-walking towards the roundabout near our house. Above us, gnarled eucalypts bend and twist like demons, making shadows in the light cast by the streetlamps.

I can't believe he said that. Or perhaps he didn't say it. Perhaps I am embellishing.

Later, my psychologist will tell me that this illness distorts my memory. She will say that it is like childbirth: the body can't go on if it remembers the wholeness of the pain. My body is invoking some ancient survival mechanism. Unable to numb the pain itself, it numbs instead my recollection of it.

Memory isn't a static thing. Each time I try to recall a memory, I am changing it, altering it. The more I write, the more I mythologise.

I want to remember how I felt, what I did, what was said, yet my memory feels elusive, like a ghost. I want to trace and retrace its paths. I could be making this worse. Perhaps I am distorting reality, seeing monsters where there are only shadows. Perhaps I am filling the gaps in my memories with fables.

My doctors speak about my illness in clinical, rational terms. I fictionalise it: spells and episodes.

1.

Our universe moves in loops and spirals. Planets rollick and spiral around stars that spin and twist along the long arms of galaxies. From Earth, where we are also spinning in orbit, spirals can appear circular, even static. We don't notice them, miss them altogether. Begin to look, and spiral shapes can be found in abundance. Water swirling down a drain, the golden ratio of a shell, the clouds of a cyclone. The spirals of space are even mirrored in the outward spiral of embryonic matter. In utero, our cells grow and multiply not in straight and linear ways, but through twisting and coiling. Our spines unfurl like ferns. The pattern of the moon loops into the pattern of the womb.

In 1492, Christopher Columbus looked out from the *Santa María* and saw the ocean alive, moving, glowing. Beneath the waves, thousands of bioluminescent worms performed their mating dance. On the nights following a full moon, worms emerge from the sediment of the ocean floor. They move in slow circles, leaving spirals of luminescent mucus in their wake. Columbus described the sight as 'the flame of a small candle alternately raised and lowered'. To the humans aboard the

Santa María, unfamiliar with this particular biological process, the worms appeared magic, or miracle.

Worms are not the only species to dance beneath the moonlight. There are nights when the Great Barrier Reef grows thick with the eggs and sperm of coral polyps, corals dancing and long-distance mating at just the right time, in sync, erupting in unison. Researchers believe that to make their moonlit rendezvous, these animals must hold within themselves not only a circadian clock, but a circalunar clock, too.

In the worst moments of the COVID-19 lockdowns, I found myself spiralling. Within my spiral, the world appeared static.

On a dark night, no moon in sight, I leave the outdoor light on. When I return to switch it off, a moth is beating itself against the glass bulb. It spins and flickers, leaving trails of wing dust, disoriented by an artificial moon.

An environment can shape a body. In old times, before streetlamps, our cycles may have followed the patterns of the moon more closely. We stayed up later on full-moon nights, slept less. The moon told us when to plant our crops, and when to harvest. It provided a metronome with which to count the days and seasons. Some researchers believe the moon may have influenced our own menstrual cycles, too. Once, for six months, I synced with the lunar calendar. Like some kind of worm or polyp, I ovulated at the full moon. My body became a circalunar clock. By causation or correlation, I was happy.

Scientists once believed that the woman whose menstrual cycle aligned with the moon was the most fertile. Now, this is largely considered woo-woo nonsense.

The summer before the lockdowns started, I ended a four-year relationship and fell hard for the rebound. I'd started to think of beginnings and endings as loops in a spiral. My ex and I had the same arguments over and over, tracing the same narrative circles again and again.

In 2006, neuroscientist Jill Bolte Taylor made an extraordinary observation: emotions only last in the body for around 90 seconds. That is to say that from feeling the emotion, to recognising it and acknowledging it, to letting it dissipate in the body is a process that only takes a minute and a half. What draws out our experience of the emotion is not the feeling itself, but the narratives we construct around it: the stories we tell ourselves. Were we able to just sit with an emotion for 90 seconds, acknowledge it without reacting to it, our bodies may let it go. When we instead start justifying and rationalising that emotion, perhaps even acting on it, we risk getting caught in a feedback loop, reigniting the physiological sensations of that emotion again and again and again. We write ourselves into spirals. Something as shifting as a story can keep us stuck.

I think of ants. Naturally blind, army ants navigate the world through scent. One ant will trace its path, leaving behind a trail of pheromones for the next to follow. Should this path become jumbled, or loop back on itself, the ants get stuck. It's called a death spiral. As more and more ants follow the scent of the pheromones before them, the death spiral grows thick, like the storm clouds of a hurricane, or stars in the Milky Way. Each ant follows the spiral, retraces the loop, lays down new pheromones until, exhausted, it drops dead.

I'd been indecisive about the break-up. I loved him, but I felt stuck. The week before we ended things, I applied to study at three overseas universities and bought a couch. I was between worlds, unsure which way to turn. I feared we would keep hurting each other in the same ways, over and over, not knowing any better.

The night I ended it, Dad picked me up.

'What'd he do?' he asked when I got in the car.

'Nothing—just, nothing.'

My ex was still inside our apartment, metres away. I'd left him lying on the bed, facedown. All the lights were off.

Dad put a hand on my shoulder and I started crying. I hate crying in front of people. It feels performative, like I'm trying to pull sympathy, whether it's due or not.

'He's unhappy,' I said.

'Unhappy with your relationship?' Dad asked.

'With the world? I don't think he can tell where one unhappiness ends and another begins.'

Dad frowned. 'There's a difference between being unhappy about the world and unhappy in a relationship. I'm sure he can tell the difference.'

I shrugged. I wasn't so sure.

—

The rebound was a friend—Pavan. At first, I was less enamoured of him than I was of my own excitement. The year of the rat was approaching, the first animal in the lunar zodiac, a time for new beginnings. I had a *crush* again. With Pavan, everything felt transitory. Under the guise of friendship, we expected little of each other.

He was camping with my friends at Meredith Music Festival, and we found each other on a couch in the early hours of the morning.

'Do you want to talk about it?' he asked. 'The break-up?'

I licked my lips. 'It's all I want to talk about. It's all I can think about.'

'We can talk about it, if you want.'

'I want nothing more—but I also don't want to be that person,' I said, stretching my legs out from under me. 'It's boring. I could talk about it for days.' The worst thing about break-up clichés was how many of them were true.

'You're talking to the perfect person, then,' said Pavan. 'I could talk about love for days.'

I asked him out the following weekend. We'd just finished a week-long clowning class together, during which he was funny, and I was mortified. He beamed at me, said he had a crush too. For a moment, I felt like nothing could hurt me. Like I was immune to heartbreak. Pavan felt like part of an ending, and then a beginning, too.

My ex kept the apartment, so I made plans to house-sit for three different people over the summer. Pavan moved into each house with me, and in each house we lived a different life. In one, we had a dog and a gas stove, and played at domestic bliss. In another, we took too many drugs and barely slept. We went for picnics in Edinburgh Gardens, had our friends over for dinner parties. We'd lived in the same orbit for years, yet this Pavan felt new: I had no preconceptions of him, no anticipation of us. We talked for hours in brick courtyards, until the city glowed orange with smoke and we moved inside. We shared stories of our past loves, our families, our fears. We forgot to eat. When we finally remembered, we cooked lavish meals for each other, pretended it was how we always did things. He joked about being vegan to impress me, then went vegan for real. I'd always known Pavan was a romantic, and now I was, too. We both liked the narrative of a summer spent wildly in love.

We'd been living together twenty-four-seven for three weeks when I told him it was too soon for anything serious.

'I know,' he said. 'I just want to watch you live.'

A few weeks later, we were walking along Brunswick Street. As we neared my old apartment, I dropped his hand.

'You should be alone for a while,' he said later, over potato cakes. He looked sadder this time.

'What do you mean?'

'It's too soon—you should be single for a bit.'

This time I picked up his hand.

'Maybe. But I'm not doing what I should do.'

I knew it was too much, too fast. We were love bombing each other, but I didn't care. I still believed myself invulnerable to hurt.

—

We spend the summer eating too many drugs and too little food. I miss my period three times over. This doesn't cause me worry: I have an IUD. I meet each missed period like a gift, an extension of summer. There, in those liminal months, time moves differently. I exist beyond its usual cycles. It is euphoria.

When summer ends, I run out of places to house-sit. My ex is in [illegible] with his work, so I spend a week crashing at my old place, watering my old plants. In the first week of March, I sign a lease on a share house in Fitzroy North, on Rae Street. It's an old terrace house with stained carpets and decades' worth of leftover furniture. It's cheap and close to the city. I tell my housemates that I won't be home much—that I'm out most nights—what with work and the month-long comedy festival coming up.

The day I sign the lease, the festival is cancelled and work goes remote. Two days later, I am accepted into a university in Las Vegas.

Pavan is in London for a wedding. I FaceTime him from my old apartment and tell him about the university.

'Sorry,' I say. 'I don't know why I'm crying. It's good news.'

Pavan looks winded, tells me he's thrilled for me.

'I'll drop you off,' he says. 'We can say goodbye with a Vegas wedding. Have a divorce party when you come back.'

I laugh. 'I'd like that.'

—

My brother helps me move my stuff from my old apartment to the new place on Rae Street. We pack my things into his Subaru and get it done in three trips. The next day, we're in lockdown.

2.

In 2015, after my first big break-up, in my early twenties, a friend and I moved into a share house in Coburg. The walls were cracked at every seam. The kitchen sloped into the ground. The house was plagued by mice who had forgotten to fear humans. It was a disease, one of our new housemates told us. *Toxoplasma gondii*, a parasite that stopped the rodents from feeling fear. They would loiter in the kitchen, strolling away—not scampering—when they saw us. We called them all Albert.

'It's only three hundred dollars a month,' I told my friend before we signed the lease. 'It has a washing machine.'

I put a limit on the number of jokes my parents were allowed to make about the state of the place.

'I live here now,' I reminded them.

The first time I took a bath in our new home, my friend handed me a glass of red wine through the kitchen–bathroom window. I thought, *I love this place.* Living there felt half terror, half magic.

We'd smoke rolled cigarettes on the front porch until we'd decide it was time to quit, then someone would buy a new pouch, and we'd start again. We traced this pattern over and over. We couldn't help ourselves.

'There's a drug called Champix,' my friend said. 'It's supposed to help you quit smoking. Something to do with dopamine. Just makes it stop feeling as good.'

We visited the bulk-billing clinic together. In the waiting room, a receptionist asked me to fill out an intake form. *Over the past two weeks, how many times have you felt down, depressed or hopeless? None of the days, some of the days, more than half of the days, nearly every day.*

My memory for moods has always been terrible. I drew loose circles down the middle.

Champix made us feel nauseous. I vomited at the corner cafe and we swore we'd never go back. We lay in my bed and watched *Orange Is the New Black*. One of the inmates, Daya, was pregnant. When she vomited, we joked that she was on Champix. *Is It Champix or Are You Pregnant?* was the name of our new game.

Nausea: Champix (and pregnant). Bloating: Champix (and pregnant). Weird dreams: Champix. You could also be pregnant.

We took the joke too far, so took turns pissing on pregnancy tests to calm our nerves.

'Two lines means not pregnant, right?' my friend asked. I thought she was joking, but she wasn't.

We went back to the doctor to make sure. The bulk-billing clinic paired her with a balding older man. He moved in a way that might have been described as leisurely but struck us as pathologically old.

'Congratulations,' he told her.

She asked him about her options, and the slowness with which he delivered his non-answers was also pathological.

When my friend called to tell her mum, she said, 'Okay. I'm at work, I can't talk right now.'

Her boyfriend was in Europe with his family. His mum booked him the earliest flight home. For a moment, I wished he wouldn't come. *This is happening to us, not him*, I thought. I didn't recognise the nastiness of my own jealousy.

My friend and I shared my bed for three nights. When her boyfriend landed at Tullamarine airport, she packed her things, then went to stay with him at his parents' house.

'I can't stay here,' she told me. 'This house feels haunted now.'

Once my friend was gone, I called my mum and let the story spill out in repetitive, nonlinear strands.

'Poor thing,' my mum said. 'I'm glad her boyfriend is with her.'

Then she helped me make an appointment to have a hormonal IUD inserted.

The doctor didn't want to do it.

'It's more likely to perforate your womb if you haven't had a kid yet,' she said. 'It could affect your fertility.'

I told her that it was fine. She worried that I would change my mind: I was 22, too young to make a decision like this. *If I am too young to make my own decisions*, I thought, *then I am too young for a child*. I told her that it was fine.

Two days later, Mum drove me to the women's clinic. Outside, anti-abortion protestors told me to think about my baby. I pictured my friend walking through that same crowd. I thought she might enjoy the theatrics.

'Count backwards from ten,' the anaesthetist told me. I got to four, blinked, woke up. I was in a hallway. At first, I thought there had been a delay, or a mistake. Then I felt a dull throb in my guts, and I realised that time had passed through me. It was over. In a waiting room down the hall, I found Mum reading a magazine.

'That was quick,' she said.

I felt terrible. In the car, I held my stomach and groaned. I asked Mum to get me water. After a sandwich and a Panadol, I was fine.

Later that afternoon, I met my friend at her boyfriend's house. It was bright, light, open. No mice, no cracks in the walls. She was on the couch, too nauseated to move. She would have to wait like that for a week. Her pregnancy had been discovered in a small window of life: too early for a surgical abortion, too late for a medical one.

'They gave me the strongest anti-nausea medication available,' she told me. 'They wouldn't let me take it if I was keeping it.'

Her boyfriend offered to cook me lunch. He had a whole adult house in front of him, a full pantry. We ate toast with peanut butter, the only thing my friend could keep down.

'I wonder if they'll let me have the foetus,' my friend said. 'I could keep it in a jar.'

My skin pricked with horror. I imagined its small embryonic spine, shrimp eyes, the mollusc shape of it. The fact that, even if it was hers, it was something else, too.

'You can't do that,' I told her.

'Why not?' she asked.

For a week, my friend was caught between universes: the one where she was pregnant, and the one where she was not. These universes were not compatible. In one, nothing changed. In the other, everything did. Within her, the two potential universes spiralled out and out.

'Look,' my friend said, then lifted her top. 'My tits are huge.'

The next morning, alone in the share house, I woke to my phone buzzing beside me. The bulk-billing clinic. 'We noticed your intake form,' they told me. 'We thought you might benefit from seeing a therapist.' I felt my head rush, like the world had been swirling around me too fast and I'd only just had the chance to notice.

The last time I'd seen a psychologist had been a year prior. I'd entered her office in tears. I could not bear to live anymore, I told her. I felt wrong, monstrous. There was something evil inside me. She suggested that I set some Specific, Measurable, Achievable, Relevant and Time-based goals, work on becoming more financially independent.

On my second visit, six weeks later, I was no longer in tears. I could hardly remember why I had cried so much in the first place.

'I'm feeling so much better,' I told her.

She smiled: 'That's great. SMART goals can really help.'

Another psychologist had mentioned schemas. She thought my feelings, recurring thoughts, patterns and behaviours were tied to some form of early childhood trauma.

I dug through my childhood looking for trauma but could only come up with the regular ones: kids being mean on the playground, not liking trips with family. I tried to stir up some resentment for the way my parents raised me—to find something they did wrong—but again, nothing.

Can the mundane be traumatic, too? I wondered. I was unsure what to believe.

'Once I cried in the car because I got a maths problem wrong,' I told the psychologist. She nodded solemnly. I left with a distrust of my memory. Was there something I had forgotten? Repressed? I spent more time analysing my feelings, trying to locate them within a time, a place, a memory, than I did actually feeling them.

I told this and more to the doctor at the bulk-billing clinic.

'It's like I'm stuck in some kind of loop,' I said. 'I feel terrible one week, the next I can hardly remember why.'

To refer me to a psychologist, the doctor needed a diagnosis. He told me that I didn't quite meet the criteria for clinical depression. Instead, he diagnosed me with premenstrual dysphoric disorder, or PMDD. He didn't know much about it and didn't take me through any formal diagnostic process, but he described the condition broadly as depression before your period. Something clicked in me. He wrote me a referral, and I left the clinic within half an hour of arriving.

At home, I googled PMDD. I couldn't find much that felt useful to me. There was a Reddit thread where people vented about their symptoms, and an academic paper debating whether the illness was real at all. Nothing solid about either a cure or a cause. I wasn't even sure which questions I should be asking: was this illness real? Did I really have it? If so, which parts of myself were me, and which were PMDD? Even though my searches came back with only thin threads for answers, I knew what was wrong. This was just the beginning but, in that moment, I thought of it as an ending. Mystery solved, life goes on.

Premenstrual dysphoric disorder. My mind and tongue tripped over the *dysphoric* part. Dysphoria, from the Greek *dys*, meaning evil, and *phoria*, to carry. An evil to carry.

3.

I move into Rae Street and everything feels temporary. *I am leaving the country soon*, I tell myself. *Don't settle down*. I don't know how to plan for anything. I don't own a bed. I sold it a year earlier, when my ex and I moved in together. I sleep on a roll-out camping mattress on the floor.

My new housemate asks that we clean and disinfect the kitchen morning and night. She wipes down the doorknobs with disinfecting wipes. Another housemate steals toilet paper from work and brings home a bucket of homemade hand sanitiser from a friend's house. I spend most days at my desk, working, and evenings at the same desk, talking to Pavan and our friends online. I feel awkward, stuck inside with four strangers. I don't tell them about the university acceptance—that I plan to move in a few months. I don't tell my work, either.

In the early weeks, we call the lockdowns 'iso', or 'quarantine', even though we're technically doing both and neither. COVID-19 has come from overseas, so the first people to actually quarantine are those from international flights. Pavan is flying back from the wedding in London and must be quarantined at home for two weeks. If he had landed a week later, he would have been put in a hotel. I can't stand it. I message my friends: *Is it worth a ten-thousand-dollar fine just to see him?* Sensibly, they tell me no.

The day he lands, I tell Pavan to get a COVID test. Not everyone's allowed to be tested yet, but he meets the criteria. Maybe, I think, a test will mean I can see him sooner.

In the group chat we share recipes for brownies, our desires to learn new skills, how we have started painting. We do YouTube workouts, give audiobook and podcast recommendations. Three weeks ago, we were sprawled over each other on couches at 4 a.m., sniffing powder from a bag. Now we're sharing housekeeping tips and meditation apps.

Pavan's COVID test comes back positive.

'I went to a wedding,' he says. 'Took an international flight.'

I imagine the virus as little spheres in his body, stampeding forward, trying to infect, infect, infect. Illness wants company.

Pavan's COVID diagnosis is, it turns out, a good thing. For me, at least. Later, we'll call it *the OG COVID*—the mild strain, just before it got crazy. His second test, only days after landing in Melbourne, is negative. Five more days and he is considered recently recovered. Bizarrely, this means that—despite having had the illness he was quarantined for—he is allowed to leave the mandatory two-week quarantine early. The day that he is released, Premier Daniel Andrews announces that lockdown restrictions are not designed to keep significant others apart.

We are allowed to visit 'intimate partners'. When we get the news, Pavan drives from his parents' house—where his family are still stuck at home, isolating as close contacts—to mine.

When he shows up at my door, I want to hug him, don't want to touch him. I think we should put him in the shower immediately, maybe burn his clothes. I don't know the protocol for this. My housemates are baffled by his arrival. They ask him what it was like and he shrugs. There have been fewer than two hundred known cases in the state, and he was one of them.

Once Pavan is in my house, I'm scared to let him leave. We're not supposed to leave anyway. But more than that, I'm scared that if he goes home, the rules will change and we'll be separated for good. I'm scared that having him over for too long will piss my new housemates off. I'm scared I'll never see him again. I'm scared he's an intrusion. I'm scared of being locked down without him. I google *cabin fever symptoms* and I'm only being a little over the top about it.

My worry directs itself outwards in strange ways. Pavan leaves his socks in the living room and I scold him for it. He makes a mess in the kitchen and I scold him for it. At night, watching TV on a laptop in the bed I'd finally caved and bought, I feel so overcome with anxiety that I start crying. We'd spent the summer living on top of one another, but this is different. I am trying to make him as unobtrusive to my housemates as possible, trying to contain him as though *he* is an illness. I can't stop pushing him around, telling him off. I snap because I am hungry, then we cook a feast for dinner, and I cry because I am too full. My emotional outbursts come on hard and unprompted.

I feel I have a dog in me. Black dog, wolf, I'm not sure. I can't remember the inciting incident, only that I grew dark, intense, moody.

After a week, I find Pavan in my room, his bag open on the end of my bed.

'I'm going home,' he tells me. There is a seriousness to his tone that stops me from arguing.

'Will you come back?' I ask.

'Of course,' he says, then packs his things to leave.

A year earlier, I had read an essay by the academic Stacy Alaimo about how rising acidity in our oceans is dissolving the shells of small marine molluscs. The spirals of their shells are being eaten away at, acid passing through to the raw flesh of their skin, now exposed.

I think of time as a spiral: the face of a clock, the circles of ancient calendars. Static within my own spiral, I curl my body into bed, imagine myself as porous as a shell, try to let time pass through me.

4.

Two days after Pavan leaves, I get my period and my body calms. I feel ashamed, embarrassed. I'd acted like a version of myself that I don't want to be.

I can't remember when this started. Perhaps it was at fifteen, when I got my first period and went on the pill. Perhaps my IUD is making it worse. I've been on and off different forms of hormonal birth control for more than a decade. When I try to remember how I used to feel, I find my memory lacking. I don't know what my baseline is; I don't know my underlying cycle. The truth is I can't remember what I am like without added hormones—the contraceptive pill, the hormonal IUD—circulating in my body, altering or masking my cycle. The IUD has made my periods lighter, but they haven't disappeared altogether. Every few months or so I skip the bleeding, but the rest of my cycle—my hormones, the moods, the irrationality—has remained the same. Or, at least, I think they have remained the same. It's hard to keep track. Perhaps my moods are worse now. I'm not sure what I was like before.

I think that perhaps I am naive, simply bad at noticing. I blur the boundaries between correlation and causation. I am the kind of person who will take a Panadol for my headache, then, when the headache goes away, think that I didn't need the Panadol after all.

With my ex, I'd spend the days before my period moody and irritable. But there was a certain roteness to my mood swings. I'd become comfortable with our cycles of arguments, and that had diverted me from better managing my own cycle. When we went to a couples counsellor, she would spend most of our sessions helping him work through his depression. My mood swings seemed like a side note.

Now, in the bright light of a new relationship, I can see which behaviours are mine and mine alone. I can see clearly the stories that I carry with me.

When I read anecdotes from other people with premenstrual dysphoric disorder, there are a few constants. People describe themselves as feeling monstrous, out of control. They feel wild, irrational, angry, manic. They fear what they may do, and fear that they are incapable of stopping it. What is missing from many of the testimonies of people with PMDD is what these people actually do. The details are sparse. They argue with their partners. They snap at the small stuff. They cry—a lot. They *feel* monstrous, but none of their actions seem *that bad*. I grow agitated reading these stories. I begin to wonder about the point at which an emotion is just an emotion, and the point at which an emotion becomes an illness, too.

—

The year after I was first diagnosed with PMDD, I read an extract from a book by Frank Bures, which argued that premenstrual syndrome is a culture-specific illness: that is, it exists only because we believe it to exist, not because it has any basis in biology. 'On the one hand,' he writes, 'we assume the causes of PMS are purely biological, despite not having found the mechanisms. And on the other we assume the causes of "cultural syndromes" are entirely mental, despite the fact that one's beliefs and expectations about a condition can generate many of the same physical symptoms.'

When Bures was researching premenstrual illnesses, science had not found a physical, or biological, cause for PMS or PMDD. This led many sceptics, including some doctors and psychologists, to view the illness as cultural. People who complained of PMS or PMDD showed no abnormal hormonal levels. It was their reaction that was abnormal.

For years, scientists could not find biological causes for depression either, until medicine caught up, and now neurological and biological causes for the condition are increasingly understood and accepted. I think of the *Santa María* and the glowing worms that must have appeared as magic to an unknowing eye: not understanding how something could exist does not mean that it can't exist at all.

I find other arguments for the cultural creation of premenstrual illness more compelling than the absence of knowledge alone. Over the past few decades, several studies have corroborated contributing factors to someone's risk of developing PMDD: childhood trauma, genetics, and—most striking to me—the *expectation* that they will have premenstrual syndrome. People who believe that PMS exists, and that it has a biological basis, experience more and worse symptoms.

When I read this, I think of how the stories we tell ourselves can keep us stuck. When we expect ourselves to be irrational, or moody, we tend to notice those states more readily. When we anticipate PMS, or PMDD, we may be quicker to rationalise our response to normal irritations—socks left out, dishes unwashed, a busy workday—as a PMS or PMDD response. In other words, people who expect to have PMS may be more likely to tell themselves a story in which their reactions to the world are abnormal.

The more ready someone is to dismiss social causes for their distress, the more intense their experience of PMS. To me, the question of whether PMDD has a biological cause is less stunning than this discovery: our culture, the stories we believe, can make an illness worse.

Bures connects the cultural myths of PMS and PMDD to other culture-specific maladies: a Nigerian illness that magics away people's genitals; Cambodian 'wind attacks', which leave people numb and breathless; *gilahari* syndrome in India, where it's believed that a lizard has crawled under the victim's skin and will kill them once it reaches their neck. Patients show up to the hospital with swelling limbs, though no lizard can be found. These illnesses, Bures argues, are as real as PMS and PMDD. The only difference is our own cultural bias: that we look for the biological causes of the illnesses we experience in our own culture and in turn dismiss or fictionalise the illnesses of other cultures.

When I first read Bures's piece, I struggle to hold two things as true. I can't understand how I can feel something so wholly, and yet at the same time be the one constructing it. I worry that I am the one turning my body against me, that I am playing the victim, that I'm just not strong enough or brave enough or resilient enough to deal with the world. I worry that I have written myself into a story where, because I am female, I am irrational and weak.

Once more, I search through my childhood, looking for answers. Once more, I come back with little.

My mother never had premenstrual mood swings. When I was small, she told me that PMS was an illness invented by men to keep women out of power. In Grade 5, Healthy Harold the Giraffe visited our primary school, taking us into his van to teach us about puberty and mood swings. Afterwards, I clutched the colourful handouts tight.

'Mum, Mum!' I said when she picked me up from school. 'Did you know that hormones make you moody? We *have* to tell Dad about this.'

Later, in high school, we said that we were PMSing when on our periods. We held our stomachs and groaned and begged our friends to fill up our water bottles for us. *Check me?* we'd ask, then flash the backs of our school dresses. We were always fine.

It feels impossible to know whether I experience PMDD because I have PMDD, or because I believe in PMDD. Growing up, most of what I thought I knew about premenstrual moods was wrong or confused. I'd thought PMS happened while *on* your period, not before. I'd thought it was like a cramp, or no big deal. I didn't connect my cycle to my moods until I was in my twenties. I don't think of myself as someone who *expects* to be miserable before my period, and yet I feel miserable. Now, with a diagnosis, perhaps I expect it too.

None of this is proof of anything. Still, it's hard to hold both as true: that my illness could be culturally constructed, and that I experience it in all its fullness. There are times when it catches me by surprise. There are times when I deny that I have it, only for the blood to come and my mood to lift. Just because an illness is culturally constructed doesn't mean that it isn't real. I'm not convinced that there is no biological basis for this illness. I want to hold multiple realities: that this illness is physical and mental and cultural, all at once.

'I have this thing,' I tell Pavan.

He came back this morning, each of us slow and cautious with the other. We're walking through Edinburgh Gardens and I'm trying to explain why I was such a bitch to live with.

'It's called premenstrual dysmorphic disorder,' I say, then correct myself. 'Sorry, I mean dysphoric. Premenstrual dysphoric disorder.' I still trip over the carrying part.

'You mean like PMS?' Pavan asks.

I say yes, because it's close enough.

I'm reluctant to show him this side of me. I find myself latching onto the duality of my illness. I'm not *me* when I'm sick. I become someone else. I'm no longer in control. It's not my fault. I can hear my own ableism in the way I describe it to him—that I'm not *crazy*, there is a biological explanation. I tell him it's a physical illness, not a mental one, though I'm not quite sure it's true.

He asks me what I've done to fix it and I flood red.

'Nothing, really,' I say. 'It's never been this bad.'

I'm not sure this is true, either. I don't tell him about the tidal moods my exes put up with. I don't tell him about the shame I feel for doing so little for so long. I don't tell him that I don't trust my memory enough to know how bad it gets. The truth is that most of the time, when I am well, I forget that I was ever unwell at all. I convince myself that I am moving on a linear path through time, not cycling through the same mess, over and over.

We leave the park and head towards Rae Street. We can see the Tramway Hotel, its front door locked shut. There's a sign out front: *Takeaway Coming Soon.*

'Maybe you should speak to someone,' Pavan says.

I'm terrified of losing him, so I promise him I will.

5.

Searching for truth between the myths, I stumble into crime scenes. In 1980, Sandie Craddock finished her shift at an East London bar. On her walk home, she attacked and killed her co-worker, seemingly without reason, stabbing her three times through the heart. The police arrested Sandie—not for the first time. She had 45 charges on her record: assault, arson, theft. In her case notes, she reads like a monster: a woman possessed. She had attempted suicide more than 25 times.

Sandie's father provided her legal team with a collection of his daughter's diaries. Her lawyers pored through these diaries, along with her criminal record and institutional reports, and plotted the events of Sandie's life like stars on a celestial map. An unusual pattern emerged. With only a small amount of variation, Sandie's crimes occurred every 29.04 days; her suicide attempts, which continued to be recorded by guards during her imprisonment, occurred every 29.55 days.

Every 29.55 days.

Every 29.53 days, the moon completes its cycle of phases. Sandie's lawyers painted her as a werewolf. They mapped her actions against a circalunar clock.

Leading up to her trial, Sandie Craddock's violence continued. She strangled another prisoner. Attempted escape. Gouged her wrists. Attacked a warden. Tried to hang herself. Every 29 days.

Sandie pleaded not guilty on account of diminished responsibility. Craddock, her lawyers claimed, suffered from premenstrual syndrome. They argued that she was not responsible for her actions—that it was automatism. She was out of control, not herself, acting on hormones rather than reason.

The key defence witness was Katharina Dalton, a physician and expert in premenstrual syndrome, a term she helped coin in the 1950s. After reading Sandie's diaries, Dr Dalton agreed with the lawyers' theory that the defendant suffered from this condition, and diagnosed her with it.

Dalton began dosing Sandie with massive amounts of progesterone. Sandie's personality changed completely. She was docile, no longer violent. Stable, even. Her 29-day cycles of violence ended.

'She knew what she was doing,' Dalton told the court. 'But she could not control herself. She lost her moral safeguards.'

Sandie's trial judge rejected any defence of automatism: 'It is quite clear from the doctor's evidence that this woman knew exactly what she was doing, intended to do it, but was led into doing it because the dark side of her nature appeared.'

Still, the jury recognised the role premenstrual syndrome played in Sandie Craddock's actions that night. Her charge was reduced to manslaughter due to diminished responsibility. She received a sentence of three years of probation, during which she would continue to receive hormone treatments. She avoided further punishment.

Missing from all the case files I read: who was the co-worker she stabbed? What was said?

I try to think back on my own actions during the premenstrual—the luteal—days of my cycle, but my memories are foggy and vague. I remember arguments, but never what they were about, what was said. I've never attacked anyone, never bit or stabbed or murdered. Still, I begin to doubt myself. I might not have hurt anyone, never seriously hurt myself, but I know I've wanted to. Perhaps I am remembering things wrong. Perhaps I'm still bad at noticing.

I start to make a list of all the things I have done while spiralling. I want to hold myself accountable, want to know what I am capable of. Once, with my ex, I felt so enraged by—*what?*—that I went for a walk, felt my body clench like a scream and punched a brick wall. My hand jarred, my knuckles stung, the wall more unyielding than I'd imagined. On another occasion, we went away for a weekend with his friends, and I was so overwhelmed with—*what?*—that I struggled to make nice conversation. While everyone else left for a day hike, I stayed behind. I made my way to the beach, stripped off my clothes and dunked my body in the freezing ocean. It was only later, noticing some fishermen on a nearby cliff, that I realised the absurdity of my actions. I snuck back to shore, dressed my clammy body in sand-strewn clothes. I once cried at work over—*what?*—then took an extra-long lunchbreak and sobbed while picking at my banh mi, considered taking the rest of the day off. Unable to articulate the cause of my distress, I instead chose to return to the office, quiet and unfocused.

In each of these moments, I knew that I needed help. But then my period came, the fog lifted and I forgot the person I had been the day before.

I hardly remember how unwell I was. I don't know how to understand this illness without remembering the whole of it.

Monsters often represent cultural fears. In his influential 1996 anthology *Monster Theory*, academic and author Jeffrey Jerome Cohen brings together a collection of essays exploring the role monsters play in mirroring the cultures that create them. In his introduction, Cohen argues that the monsters we see on screen reflect the anxieties of their times. Usually, these monsters are born from a point of difference: a fear of the other. 'For the most part,' Cohen writes, 'monstrous difference tends to be cultural, political, racial, economic, sexual.' The creation of monsters, then, is a way to assert borders, a way to distinguish between *us* and *them*.

In 1981, the year that Sandie Craddock went to trial, three major film releases featured werewolves: *The Howling*, *An American Werewolf in London* and *Wolfen*. Like Sandie's trial proceedings, these films painted a picture of humanity's dark nature.

The Howling tells the story of Karen, a journalist who, after a close encounter with a serial-killer-slash-rapist, is sent to a place called the Colony—a New Age retreat—to process her trauma. Of course, the Colony has a secret. It is filled with werewolves.

The Howling was a reaction to the hippie, free-loving 1960s and '70s. By the 1980s, the New Agers and freethinkers had given way to actual monsters: Charles Manson, Jim Jones. Fake radicals who exploited the movement for their own gain. The Manson murders and Jonestown had turned the New Age movement into a violent spectre. Sexual liberation became sexual deviancy. Drug experimentation turned into drug addiction. In this light, *The Howling*'s werewolves represent the ideals of free love and free thought descending into animal depravity.

'We should never try to deny the beast—the animal within us,' claims the Colony's founder, Dr George Waggner. Within the Colony, animal impulse is the natural order of things. Virtue is lost; sex and violence are found. Karen's husband is bitten, then seduced into infidelity. While investigating, Karen encounters the man who caused her to be sent to the Colony in the first place—first in his human form, then as a wolf. She flees but is also bitten. Soon she will be overcome by animal desire, her human morals lost. Unable to avoid her fate, she rushes to the newsroom where she works. She speaks directly to camera:

> The day we are born, there is a battle we must fight: a struggle between what is kind and peaceful in our natures, and what is cruel and violent. That choice is our birthright as human beings, it is the real gift that differentiates us from the animals. It is as natural to us as the air we breathe, and yet all of us take it for granted. But now for some of us, that choice has

> been taken away. A secret society exists and is living among all of us. They are neither people, nor animals, but something in between. Monstrous mutations whose violent natures must be satisfied.

In *The Howling*, werewolves signify a loss of control, an inability to check our cruellest instincts. With a howl, Karen transforms into a werewolf on a live broadcast, showing the world the truth of her words. The message is simple and horrific: we must fear our natural impulses, rein them in, or risk becoming the unimaginable.

Like the werewolves at the Colony, Sandie Craddock was driven by animal instinct, per the defence narrative crafted by her lawyers. Her crimes were monstrous mutations—brief concessions to the dark side of her nature. She was a woman, and women are not meant to be violent. According to Katharina Dalton, progesterone made Sandie 'sensible and docile', while without it, a 'hidden animal' was released. She was not thinking, only acting on impulse.

There is a certain dualism that underlies Sandie's defence of automatism. Automatism: an action carried out without thought or control. I think of the Cartesian divide between the thinking man and the unthinking animal. The body acting alone, without thought or reason. This is the legacy of mathematician and philosopher René Descartes, who conceived of the mind and the body as two distinct entities, the former belonging solely to man, the latter a non-thinking entity, machine-like in its function. When the judge told Sandie that she was acting on 'the dark side of her *nature*', she was made to be less human—less responsible, but also less whole. Since the seventeenth century, this Cartesian divide of mind and body has served to dehumanise women and de-animalise animals—to sever living beings into categorisable components and reinforce a patriarchal hierarchy. Man, then woman, then animal. Though science has complicated much of Cartesian thinking—an animal is not a machine, and a human is also a kind of animal—these hierarchies are slower to come tumbling down.

Sandie Craddock's defence illustrates these themes and hierarchies. She is too close to nature to be thinking. She is somehow less mind, more body. She is less human, more animal.

In the months and years following Sandie's trial, sections of the legal world erupted in debate over the premenstrual defence. Was it a fair way to accommodate for mental illness, or was it simply an excuse for women to get away with murder? In a culture that fears deviance from the norm, it seems impossible to hold two things as true: that women are human, and are thinking, rational beings; and that women can experience a particular distress that causes them to act in humanly irrational ways.

To me, the depiction of Sandie-the-monster feels too reductive. Her humanity has been lost amid the noise of her crimes and the patterns of the moon. In her case notes, she reads less as an individual woman and more as a vessel for all the cultural anxieties surrounding women at the time: that women's involvement in work would disrupt family structures, that they can be evil and manipulative, that they are irrational and uncontrolled; or—alternatively—as a vessel for the feminist anxiety that women will continue to be patronised and met with paternalism when they, as whole humans, do terrible, human things.

If I am honest, narratives of female monsters appeal to me because I have always felt that I am a bit *too much*. Too emotional, too demanding, too dramatic. I can be lazy and impulsive. I want too much and give too little. I am angry, unthinking, perhaps out of control. I, too, am overloading Sandie with my own fear. I turn inwards to try to understand my own anxieties, to try to look at the parts of myself that I have always found a little monstrous.

Once, on a particularly unpleasant day when I was in a particularly unpleasant mood, a man cut me off while I was walking onto an escalator. My body stiffened, my throat tightened. I was too aware of my hot face, whiplash limbs, the pulse in my neck. The escalator crawled, each second lengthened by agitation. Finally, at the top, I rushed forward to overtake him—then stopped abruptly. He toppled over me, swearing. I think I smiled.

If I have not hit anyone, it is not because I have not wanted to. I feel like I have the capacity to hurt or damage or maim. Mostly this has been directed at myself or at the inanimate: a door slammed too hard, a kick to a shut gate, a slap to my own forehead. Perhaps I, like Sandie, am capable of monstrosities.

Mid-March, outside Piedimonte's Supermarket, someone has spray-painted blue footprints at metre-and-a-half intervals. Pavan and I wait on individual footprints as a staff member lets people in one at a time.

Halfway through the queue, the human footprints beneath me turn canine. Someone has painted a pair of dog paws. It's cute.

'Anyone talking about the fact there's a werewolf in this store right now?' Pavan jokes.

The line moves forward and the prints turn human once more.

Most lycanthrope—or werewolf—depictions are male: a man suffering from a Jekyll-and-Hyde-like severing of the self. There is the human side—rational, placid, sensible—and the wolf side: animal, violent, sense-seeking.

I start searching for monsters written by women and find them in the early 2000s, when masculine werewolf tropes took a feminine turn. In the Canadian film *Ginger Snaps* (2000), a werewolf attacks Ginger on the night of her first period, attracted by the scent of her blood. Within days, Ginger is overwhelmed by simultaneous symptoms of puberty and lycanthropy. When she complains to the school nurse of muscle cramps, bleeding, mood swings and hair in new places, the nurse dismisses her concerns, saying these are normal parts of becoming a woman. The *Charmed* episode 'Once in a Blue Moon' (2004) opens with its three sister-heroines eating ice cream and bemoaning PMS, only to later turn into literal fanged monsters under the light of a blue moon. When confronted with their demonic actions, the sisters write it off as 'that time of the month'. The 1999 film *The Curse* is said to be inspired by Sandie Craddock's trial. The bitten protagonist, Frida, tracks her wolf symptoms like I track my period. Formerly vegetarian, she begins to crave meat. She wakes to find her lovers dead. She complains to her doctor about PMS, and he tells her it's all in her head. The horror Frida inflicts is loaded in feminist irony: 'the curse', it turns out, is real.

Australian werewolf scholar and psychotherapist Chantal Bourgault du Coudray sees the conflation of werewolves and menstruation as 'an obvious theme for stories about female lycanthropy'. She argues that the cultural connections between lunar and menstrual cycles create neat parallels for stories of female embodiment—perhaps more so than those of male werewolves. While many of these stories are celebratory or even 'a source of personal empowerment', they often restate the ways in which female bodies can become sites of cultural anxiety and disgust. Menstruation turns women into monsters. The non-menstruating self becomes the menstruating other. An animal, a bitch. In horror, as in menstruation, the female body is abject.

There's a seductive analogy between puberty and werewolf transformation: both feature uncontrollable urges, changing bodies, a blurring boundary between human and animal impulse. Suddenly hair where previously none. Suddenly prone to animal instinct; to biting and lashing out. It's a neat comparison, but one that also reinforces certain biological tropes when applied to women: that to be a woman is to be monstrous, that menstruation is a curse. As professor of cinema Aviva Briefel argues, 'the menstruating monster exposes her biological identity with every drop of blood she sheds, both her own and her victim's'.

In works of horror, female rage can seldom be suppressed. It erupts in monstrous form. There is power in this: power in a monstrous woman's ability to be more instead of less. Yet with this power comes punishment. Become too much and become a monster. As I watch each woman transform on screen, each a victim of her own biology or monstrous mutation, I don't feel the empowerment of female rage, but instead the inevitability of it. When these women become wolves—literal embodiments of PMS bitches—there's some irony in the fact that everyone tells them it's fine, *it's normal*, when really it's not. The truth is that few women know what is normal when it comes to their cycles. The norm is to expect women to suffer.

From 1978 to '82, researchers in India observed crime rates across three different towns. They mapped their data against the movements of the moon and found that crime was more common on nights when the moon was full. 'The increased incidence of crimes on full moon days may be due to "human tidal waves" caused by the gravitational pull of the moon,' the researchers wrote.

No other studies have been able to mimic these results. This myth—that a full moon causes heightened crime—is just that: myth. The results of the study are either fluke or bias, but the ideas evoked linger in our cultural consciousness.

Humans have long made superstitious connections between the movements of the moon and the tides of human behaviour. As I try to trace the lineage of these moon myths—tangential lines that may or may not intersect—I find myth melding into myth, like old wives' tales. One theory is that, before artificial light, more people left their homes during the full moon simply because they could see better. They stayed out later, slept less, got into more drama. This correlation led us to blame the moon for our own erratic behaviour. Another theory: our belief in lunacy is simply bias, or selective memory. We are more likely to remember unusual events if they align with phenomena like a full moon. And another: people once truly believed that werewolves prowled under the full moon, then, when rationalism and disbelief settled in, the myth changed; the wolves became people, acting out under the same moon. A myth based on a myth, that wolves howl at the moon. In truth they howl for each other, whether the moon is there or not.

When Sandie Craddock was on high doses of progesterone, she was calm, rational, controlled. I think of the saying *between a wolf and a dog*. In a certain kind of light, during those twilit or moonlit hours, it's impossible to tell the difference between a wolf and a dog, the known and unknown.

I consume these stories of monsters and wolves because I am afraid that I am a monster. I can see the too-neat parallels between my monthly spirals and the lycanthrope. I hate the inevitability of it, the predictable nature of something so wholly out of my control. I cringe away from these menstrual allegories at the same time as I am drawn to them. What keeps me coming back to these monsters are their expressions of anger: how at a time when women are so ridiculed, belittled, reduced, horror maintains a space for female rage. Within this space, these women can abandon the boundaries of their bodies and be transformed into something other—something monstrous, sure, but powerful, too. I feel like I am picking at scabs. I want to be angry, want to be powerful, but am afraid of the horror that follows.

6.

Pavan and I move between my place and his parents' house. We're manic, stir-crazy. Online, people share their lockdown projects: paintings, sourdough, novels, home renos. Bunnings is still open, so we decide to redo his childhood bedroom. He drops hundreds of dollars on green paint and wooden shelves. We spend the weekend painting his room, then binge-watch comedy specials in bed, high on paint fumes.

For a moment, everything is perfect again. Pavan cooks and cleans. I write and paint. The world is stunning. I forget about the mood swings. I am somewhere between the edge of depression and the cusp of escape. I imagine myself coming out of lockdown hot and skinny, with a manuscript in tow.

Each morning, we tune in to ABC news and watch the updates. Each morning, Premier Daniel Andrews appears in his North Face jacket to report on the number of new cases. The curve is flattening. Each morning, we hope for better news, the end of this lockdown, the ability to see our friends again.

I am bored. Wildly bored.

Work feels repetitive, dull, pointless. I work in comms: social media, website management, any assortment of comms-adjacent tasks. My workplace has started releasing COVID-19 fact sheets, with updates on the restrictions and laws each time they change. It's now my job to update the website with each new change. Stay-at-home orders are in place. You may only leave your house to seek medical attention, acquire groceries, exercise outdoors or visit someone in need of medical attention. Masks must be worn in public. Restaurants can serve takeaway only. We're allowed to walk outside with one other person, one metre apart. Then we're not. For a moment, Pavan and I jokingly start to plan our wedding, then I update the fact sheets to reflect the new rules: all weddings are banned.

The American university messages me about my plans to move in August. I update the website to reflect that all international travel is banned. Australian citizens must apply for emergency exemptions to leave the country. Death, sickness, family crisis. Slowly it dawns on me that I am not going to the United States in August.

I feel caged, stuck, complacent.

It could be worse. Online, I see people across the world getting sick, dying, screaming at each other about masks. At least here there is a sense of collective purpose. We're all in it together. I don't fear getting COVID: I am only bored.

The Monday after we paint Pavan's room, I spend the morning editing a COVID fact sheet, only for more changes to come through. I scrap it and start over. Across from me, Pavan alternates between working on a new screenplay idea and playing the drums. I grow resentful.

'Come on,' says Pavan. 'Let's go for a walk.'

I message my boss that I am taking lunch, and Pavan and I start walking through the suburban blocks of Bundoora. Halfway through the walk, I remember an email that I forgot to reply to and feel a panic coming on.

'Relax,' says Pavan.

The way he says it reminds me of my ex, how he would say, *Relax, it's just your anxiety*, whenever I moved too quickly, be it with stress, nerves or excitement.

'Don't tell me to relax,' I snap, and I am immediately embarrassed at myself.

For decades, most of our understanding of dog behaviour came from observations of wolves in captivity. In the wild, wolves have complex social dynamics. In captivity, these dynamics are muddied by human intervention, shrunken territories, unrelated wolves being forced to live together. In captivity, wolves show more aggressive and dominant behaviour than they do in the wild. Here is the myth of the alpha: one wolf leads the pack. In the wild, social hierarchies are less rigid.

As humans, we have observed wolves in captivity and superimposed the resulting theories onto wild wolves. We have assumed that a wolf in a cage is a wolf is a dog.

From my bedroom, in lockdown, I try to unpack my own behaviour. I am irritable, irrational—aggressive, even. I continue to snap at Pavan without thinking. I'm running on reflex or instinct—whose reflex or instinct, I'm not sure.

Pavan is stronger than me, but even he is wearing thin.

I make an appointment with an old therapist, tell her about the PMDD.

'I'm not sure how to help with that,' she says. 'It seems like a biological issue.'

I tell her that I'm not sure what to do, either. She talks me through some relaxation exercises. In one, I am supposed to count five things I can see, four things I can hear, three things I can feel, two things I can smell and one thing I can taste. I spend the rest of the evening swilling spit around my mouth, trying to notice what my tongue tastes like.

On the last day of March, we're set up in the living room, watching *Tiger King* on a laptop. I'm irritable, but it feels like a rational kind of irritable. We've been fighting about the dishes. By that, I mean I've been fighting. He keeps promising to do them, and then leaving them out overnight. I'm pulling my hair out, begging him either to *just do them* or to tell me that he won't, so I can get them done.

'It's not fair on my housemates,' I say. 'I'm going to do them.'

'No, no, no,' Pavan says. 'I'll do them now.'

He nudges me back onto the couch, then clatters around the kitchen. I feel itchy, impatient. I also feel right.

Undermining my righteousness is the fact that I have been fighting, in some way, all day. I have been crying, too. I cried on our walk to get coffee. I turned my camera off and cried during my morning Teams meeting. I cried when Pavan kissed me on my lunchbreak. I cried on my run after work. I cried when I got home, when Pavan asked me what was wrong and I could not grasp any specific thing that was wrong, and that seemed wrong enough to cry over.

But now I am not crying, and I can see clearly what is wrong: the dishes.

What is the point of having a partner help, I wonder, *if it takes this much mental energy*?

By this point, it feels like I have done the dishes five times over, just by how much we've talked about it. I take a breath, try to relax.

Pavan plops back down on the couch next to me.

'Done,' he says. 'See? Easy.'

'Thank you,' I say. I'm still tense, still cranky.

We hit play on *Tiger King* and I find myself rubbed all wrong about it. There are too many tigers in cages, there is too much glorified animal exploitation. Everyone hates Carole Baskin, and even though the narrative of the TV show is supposed to explain why, it still feels like misogyny to me. I can't bring myself to love Joe Exotic and hate her.

On screen, a tiger walks back and forth in front of a metal fence. I feel the same impulse to pace. I get up to grab myself a glass of water.

'Next episode?' Pavan asks.

In the kitchen, the pots and pans in the drying rack still have scabs of food around their rims. I feel my chest deflate, my head pulse.

'Fucking hell,' I say. 'You didn't clean the pots properly.'

I pick the dirty ones out of the drying rack and put them back into the sink, run the hot water.

'I can do it,' Pavan says.

'I already am,' I say. I'm done with the back-and-forth. I just want them done and done properly. If I have to think about the dishes for a second longer, I will go insane. I already feel insane. I am struck silly by what Helen Garner calls 'the insane rage of the person who does all the housework', and I don't even do that much housework. Still, I know the rhetoric of this argument. I view my rage as gendered. Online, they have words for this: weaponised incompetence, strategic incompetence, mental load, etc, etc. I feel heart-hurt over dishes and just want it to stop.

When I'm done, I sit back down on the couch with a huff.

'Another episode?' Pavan asks again, quietly this time.

'I don't think I can do another episode right now,' I say. 'Something else.'

'Whatever you think,' Pavan mumbles.

'*Buffy*?' I suggest. He doesn't say anything. I'm talking to a brick wall. 'Or should we just go to bed?'

'Sure,' he says. He shuts the laptop in a way that is clearly sulky, and I feel more irritated than sympathetic.

We lie down in the bedroom and I'm still wired. I know I have been too much, too often, but for once I don't feel out of control in my anger. I feel justified. Pavan lies next to me. His silence is obnoxious, loud.

'We can watch another episode if it's that important to you?' I say.

He says nothing.

'Look, I'll put it on.'

I take his laptop, open Netflix. He takes it back off me, shuts it down again.

'What is your problem?' I ask. 'I'm sorry I don't want to watch *Tiger King*, okay?'

'It's not about *Tiger King*,' he says.

'Then what?'

He turns his body away from me. 'I don't want to talk about it.'

I know he wants me to fish the truth out of him—to guess what it's really about—but I'm tired, frustrated, can't be bothered.

'Fine,' I say, and roll over. Our silence carries weight. I'm no good at sitting with it. After a moment, I roll back around to face him.

'Come on,' I say. 'Tell me what's up.'

Finally, Pavan relents.

'I'm just trying to think of the words for it,' he says. 'I feel bad.'

'Is it something I said? About *Tiger King*?'

'No,' he says. 'Before that.'

I'm lost. I try to coax it out of him, and eventually he's able to tell me that it's not about *Tiger King* at all, but about the dishes. That he knows he did them wrong, but he didn't mean to. He says that the way I spoke to him made him feel small, like a failure. That he doesn't quite know how to talk about it because he knows he's in the wrong, but in that moment, the shame makes him want to run.

'Right,' I say.

'I don't like when you swear at me. It's not nice.'

'I didn't swear at you,' I say.

'You did. About the pots.'

He's right. I want to explain that I wasn't swearing *at* him, that I was just frustrated, but the difference is minuscule. Instead, I tell him that I'll try to be better. It's a promise that leaves me lopsided. I can try to be better, but I don't quite know which parts of me are wrong.

'I'm trying, too,' he says.

7.

I live to go to the supermarket. Outside of home and the park, it's the only place we're allowed to go. At the self-serve check-out, I strongly consider scanning and paying for each item individually, just to make the tiny hit of dopamine I get from each purchase stretch longer.

When my cycle loops around again and I realise that I am truly, properly depressed, I order bottles of cheap prosecco online to send as anonymous gifts to my friends. I place the order from my bedroom floor, wearing the same pyjamas I've been sitting in for three days straight.

'You don't have to do that,' Pavan says.

'It's my money.'

'So buy something for you, then.'

He doesn't know that this is calculatedly, selfishly, just for me. It costs me $81.60: more than I would spend on myself. But now, not only do I get the dopamine hit from buying something, but also the dopamine of waiting for my friends to realise that they have received a gift, the dopamine when they message me to tell me about it, and the dopamine of knowing that, even if I cannot make myself happy, I can make someone else happy for just a little while.

The results are exponential. With six bottles, I reach ten friends across six addresses. I am an expert at microdosing happiness, a fiend for dopamine.

My work routine falters. When Pavan is over, he sleeps late. I work on COVID-19 fact sheets until he stirs, copy-pasting text from a Word document into WordPress, then fiddling around with the code. I'm jealous of his slowness, the way he wakes with no alarm, then stretches and lounges for a while before finally rising.

Once Pavan is up, we go on our coffee walk—the highlight of my day. Three cafes near us serve takeaway coffee through their windows, and we alternate between them for a little variety. If I'm lucky, I won't have another meeting for a while, and we'll walk through the park with our coffees, my phone in my hand so I can pretend to be at my desk if anyone calls.

Pavan watches the morning news while I work. Case numbers are falling, slowly, slowly. Five new cases can ruin our morning. A doughnut day—zero cases—can make it.

On good days, I power through as many fact sheets as I can, make graphics for social media, write newsletters about the effectiveness of our COVID response. None of it feels right, none of it feels good enough. On bad days, I stare at my screen, retyping the same email again and again, neither productive nor relaxed.

Most of the good days are spent making up for the bad days. I feel myself slowly slipping. I worry that I will never catch up. I start doing work at strange hours, out of guilt or necessity, I'm not sure.

I look up the symptoms of burnout. I have them all but tell myself I am being dramatic. I hardly work enough to be burnt out.

When Pavan is at his parents' house, I feel aimless.

I rearrange my room, then rearrange it again a day later. On the news there's talk of restrictions easing, until six new cases at a meat-processing facility put an end to hope. Six grows to a dozen, then close to a hundred. Soon there are more than a thousand active cases in the state. I joke-text Pavan that it's just another reason to go vegan, but the anger I feel is deep and hopeless.

On a Tuesday afternoon, I call him in tears. I feel the very definition of *hysterical*. I ask if he can come over. When he asks me what's wrong, I give no answer, only ugly, gasping sobs. When he arrives, I'm a grateful, apologetic mess.

'It would be an issue if you weren't self-aware,' he says after the crying stops. 'But you are.'

I know what he means, but I take little comfort in it. I feel that were I just a little more self-aware, a little more in control, I wouldn't call him crying in the first place. If I were a little more self-aware, I would remember what the tears had been about afterwards.

Later that night, I dream that I am repotting the smallest of my plants. I brush the dirt away from its roots slowly and carefully. It is a measured, delicate act of care.

On days off, I lie in bed with Pavan until I can't stand the stillness. I try to write, get twenty thousand words into a novel before I realise it's a short story, and cut it down to three thousand. I focus on painting instead: oils. I've never used them before. I paint deranged portraits of myself and Pavan. My parents' dog, too. After two weeks, I put the paintbrushes down and don't pick them up again.

Pavan, who writes for TV, decides that he wants to write prose. He's obsessed with David Sedaris and shares his views on stretching the truth in service of the story. We spend a day working on flash stories for an upcoming deadline. Pavan's is accepted first, and I feel a sour kind of happy. Then my own acceptance letter comes through an hour later and I breathe a sigh of relief, suddenly aware of how close I am to the edge of something.

8.

After giving birth to her child, the narrator of *The Yellow Wallpaper* (1892) suffers a nervous episode. Her husband, John, is a physician, and does not believe her when she tries to describe how truly rotten she feels.

'If a physician of high standing,' she writes, 'and one's own husband, assures friends and relatives that there is really nothing the matter with one but temporary nervous depression—a slight hysterical tendency—what is one to do?'

Her brother, also a physician, and the other men in her life do not believe her when she describes her pain. Nothing is physically wrong with her; nothing is wrong with her.

She takes tonics, air, exercise, and is forbidden from working.

'Personally, I disagree with their ideas.

'Personally, I believe that congenial work, with excitement and change, would do me good.'

She becomes preoccupied with the wallpaper in her bedroom, where she is confined most days. It is a sickly, ghastly yellow. Torn in places. The pattern is ugly, darting off at odd angles. It's both confusingly dull and egregiously varied in its design. 'There is a recurrent spot where the pattern lolls like a broken neck and two bulbous eyes,' she writes. When she tells her husband about how hideous she finds the wallpaper, he laughs.

'I get unreasonably angry with John sometimes,' she writes. 'I never used to be so sensitive. I think it's because of this nervous condition.'

Charlotte Perkins Gilman wrote *The Yellow Wallpaper* in the late nineteenth century, during the Gothic Revival, which featured a renewed appreciation for haunted and supernatural aesthetics, within claustrophobic, near-medieval settings. There were female werewolves in the art of this time, too. In the literature of the Victorian and Edwardian eras, female werewolves represented the societal fear of a woman's less evolved nature, her animal instinct. These werewolves were often privileged women, women like the narrator of *The Yellow Wallpaper*. Perhaps painting these women as vicious wolves was meant as a critique of the moral degeneracy of a greedy upper class; perhaps it was born from a societal fear of a woman having power of her own.

It was only at the very end of the nineteenth century, with the rise of psychoanalysis, that the werewolf came to more closely represent 'the beast within': a shadow self, a symbolic severing of the animalistic nature that humankind should rise above, should repress.

The werewolf is a severing of selves: the human self, the wolf self. Good and evil.

I'm drawn back to the difference between a wolf and a dog. A wolf is not a domestic thing; how much more monstrous a woman's transformation, in allowing her to transcend the domestic domain.

—

Within our own four walls, I become increasingly preoccupied with the small stuff. I hate the ugly sofa in the living room. It's too big, too old, stained with who-knows-what from who-knows-who. I ask my housemates if they will let me rearrange the living room and they tell me to have at it, sceptical that anything can be done. They're right. No matter how I arrange things, the couch is still too big, too gross, and nothing fits right.

I move the furniture back to its original position. I decide the problem is that the room is too dirty. All around me I see evidence of years' worth of share-house air and share-house hygiene. Near the kitchen, it looks like oil has risen to the ceiling and dripped down the walls.

How haven't I noticed this earlier? I wonder.

I grab a bucket, a sponge, all the cleaning products in the house, and begin to scrub the walls. The water drips yellow and brown. The walls get dirtier before they get clean. It's really, really bad. I think no one must have cleaned these walls in years.

Pavan comes out of the bedroom and finds me damp and sweaty, standing on the couch in an attempt to reach the ceiling.

'What are you doing?' he asks.

'I'm cleaning the walls,' I tell him, my voice full of purpose. Afterwards, I scrub the hallways and the kitchen, too.

As the narrator of *The Yellow Wallpaper*'s maddened state nears frenzy, so does her obsession with the wallpaper. She lies in her nailed-down bed, staring at the wallpaper, following the aimless lines of its pattern for hours. She becomes determined to follow the pattern, to draw some conclusion from the senselessness of it all.

She starts to love the wallpaper: its hideousness becomes the only thing of interest in her day. When the moonlight hits the wall, the bulbous eyes in the wallpaper feel real. She believes there is a woman trapped within the wallpaper, and if she could only touch her, she could release this woman from her prison.

When no one notices how clean the walls are, I am disappointed. I feel silly. I tell Pavan that he needs to pay more attention, to notice things like the walls getting dirty, as though it's his fault that no one has noticed the walls in years. These are the fights Pavan and I have: petty arguments, pointless ones. There are times when, afterwards, I wish I wasn't quite so good at arguing. There comes a point where we are no longer fighting about the pointless thing anymore but fighting to win, to reach some conclusion.

Within the yellow-wallpapered room, the narrator's confinement becomes maddening. She begins to see the woman in the wallpaper elsewhere, too. 'I think the woman gets out in the daytime!' she writes. She sees her in the courtyard, among the roses, in every window. Her depression turns manic. She looks better, healthier. Externally, she is recovering. Internally, she is obsessed. She must release this phantom woman from the wallpaper. The wallpaper!

By moonlight, she sees the woman shaking that awful pattern. The narrator starts tearing at the walls. She rips off strips of wallpaper. She moves all the furniture around, trying to reach the room's corners. She locks the bedroom door, throws the key from the window.

When her husband returns home, he pounds at the door, tries to find an axe. When he breaks through he finds her yellow and dishevelled, rubbing herself against the walls. He faints, and she continues to crawl around the room, believing herself to be the woman in the wallpaper, finally escaped.

Gilman wrote *The Yellow Wallpaper* while undergoing her own 'rest cure'. After the birth of her daughter, she suffered from postnatal depression, for which her doctor, Silas Weir Mitchell, prescribed bed rest and a total ban on working, including reading, writing and painting. After writing *The Yellow Wallpaper*, Gilman sent a copy to Mitchell. Gilman later claimed that, though he never replied, Mitchell changed his approach to treatment after reading her story. This may have been an ecstatic dream: Mitchell continued to prescribe the rest cure and even attempted to open entire hospitals dedicated to rest. (The condescending Sir William Bradshaw in Virginia Woolf's *Mrs Dalloway*, who wants to send Septimus to a 'delightful home' in the country, is said to be based on Mitchell.)

When Gilman wrote *The Yellow Wallpaper*, the medical establishment was starting to understand hysteria less as an illness rooted in the physical—a uterine illness, as Hippocrates described it—and instead as something closer to a malady of the psyche. In 1880, the French physician Jean-Martin Charcot applied a modern scientific lens to hysteria. He believed that it was caused by some form of internal injury, which affected the nervous system. (Mitchell and Charcot met once or twice in Paris, and influenced each other's work.) One of Charcot's medical students, Sigmund Freud, took this further, defining hysteria as an entirely psychological illness. He believed that this psychological scarring emerged from an 'Oedipal moment of recognition': the moment in which a woman realises that her penis is missing. She is castrated, impotent. Though Freud theorised a psychological cause for hysteria, the connection is still physical. Women are scarred because they are not men: a person without a penis is lacking.

This was not Freud's first theory of hysteria. Before developing his Oedipal theory, he believed that his hysterical patients were victims of sexual abuse, usually at the hands of their fathers. He later repudiated this theory, unwilling to blame men when 'surely such widespread perversions against children are not very probable'. While many of Freud's patients were women, it was often their fathers who paid the bills. I take a leap and imagine that, instead of confronting these men, he chose to dismiss his hysterical patients' talk of sexual abuse as fantasy.

Today, the term *hysteria* is inextricable from the sexist connotations and treatments that surrounded it during its peak. To investigate hysteria in earnest is laughably unserious at best, and dangerously misogynistic at worst. To me, Gilman's story feels archaic. I wonder if, in another decade or two, or ten, my own experience will feel archaic, too.

—

I see my psychologist infrequently. She still doesn't know what to do about PMDD other than talk. She reminds me of this at the start of each session, and I remind her that I don't know of anyone else who can help, either. Most sessions we run through relaxation strategies: exercise, meditation, self-care.

One session, I show up fully luteal. We try to talk, but I won't stop crying. Throughout the session, I feel like I am watching myself from a distance. I see my wet face shrunken and pixellated by Zoom and feel absurd to myself. My therapist reminds me that she is not a specialist in PMDD, and I just cry. She tells me again that I likely need medication, since this is a biological issue, and I just cry. The part of me that is watching from a distance acknowledges that this is awkward, all the crying when she is clearly uncomfortable, and it would be more sensible to stop.

'I think that if I were able to leave the house, it would be better,' I say.

'Did it ever use to be this bad?' she asks.

I still don't know how to answer. I struggle to delineate the boundaries between what is normal and what is illness. I have felt this way at work, I am sure. But being in a public space, where I'm obliged to follow social conventions, sometimes allows me to mask it. Even if I mask it poorly—I've been told I have a ferocious resting bitch face—being around other people can, for a moment, jolt me out of the cycle. For moments, I forget about how *I* am feeling and instead engage with the world.

Now my only spaces are domestic. There is no reason to mask. Everything feels a little harder, and the tides of my moods are all-consuming. Has it always been this bad?

My therapist and I try to think of ways of forgetting. Activities, meditations. We both know it's hopeless.

Later in life, when asked why she wrote *The Yellow Wallpaper*, Gilman answered: 'It was not intended to drive people crazy, but to save people from being driven crazy, and it worked.' Gilman's hope was that by showing how maddening her experience of the rest cure was, she could save other women from a similar fate.

Gilman's narrator is driven mad by a patriarchal system that demands she doesn't think, doesn't feel her internal world; a system that is fearful that if she does think, she might become a problem.

Each month, I cannot tell whether what I feel is real, or whether I am being driven crazy. I am no longer able to handle the small stuff. I cry over little inconveniences. Everything stacks up. I am in lockdown, an untenable state. I am dating a man who cannot wash a dish properly. But I am not on bed rest. I am not dying. I am not any of the number of worse things that could be happening to me.

I feel that there are two halves of me: one half that can cope with these unprecedented times, and another half that cannot. In one world, I can get up, go for a walk, write three pages, put away last night's dishes, go to work, stretch, meditate, repeat. The other version of me sees a dish out in the morning and completely melts down, does nothing for the rest of the day but cry. I have honestly lost sight of which reaction is more rational.

I don't know whether it is my biology that is betraying me, or whether I am telling myself a biological myth in order to make the world seem more sane.

Some days I feel justifiably upset, only to bleed soon after. My IUD has not stopped my cycles, but they are erratic, unpredictable. I start to wonder whether I am actually luteal, or if I'm just a mess.

In my journals, my non-PMDD self appears more deranged than my PMDD self. In one entry, I am angry, frustrated, wanting to disappear. I wish I could sleep through PMDD, knock myself out. I feel horrible in my body, want to claw my skin off. *I think my IUD is making me crazy*, I write. I want to stop existing. These are the slowest quickest months on record.

In the next entry, once my period has started, I admonish myself for getting so worked up. *If I get that stressed again*, I write, *I should try a simple yoga flow.*

Days blur together and I find myself tracking my period poorly or not at all. I feel blown sideways by my emotions when they strike, and know that I'm still not doing enough to change them.

Online, women share the diets they rely on to cope with PMDD. One woman posts a TikTok of herself lounging blissfully on a crochet-covered couch, captioned: *When she fasts in ovulatory, doesn't drink caffeine in luteal, and eats omegas when she's bleeding.* I feel a flash of something hot when I see it, like maybe she's right, but I'm so annoyed by this new checklist of things to do that I want her to be wrong.

I research herbs and foods that might help, but it leaves me feeling exhausted. Outside of the luteal phase, I try to eat leafy vegetables, healthy fats, cut out sugar. But when the bad moods strike, that all falls away. I'm not convinced there's any point to it all. It seems like just another diet; another way for women to reduce, reduce, reduce, to turn their monstrous rage into something that can be controlled, portioned off and safely consumed.

On good days, I journal with optimism: *I feel so much stronger in my body! I'm eating well!* But it does little to alter the bad days that follow. It just gives me a new way to punish myself: perhaps if I were just a little more controlled, had a little more willpower, I wouldn't be so angry.

9.

I'm in that phase of my cycle and I'm telling Pavan that we need to break up.

'Is this the PMDD thing?' he asks. I feel restless, anxious, like something—anything—needs to change, and that breaking up might just be the answer. The answer to what, I'm unsure.

'Just because I'm upset doesn't mean it's my period,' I say. 'Don't use that against me.'

Pavan holds his hands in front of him as though trying to calm a bull.

'Okay, okay,' he says. 'I'm just trying to understand.'

When my period comes three days later, I'm too embarrassed to feel relief. It's so obvious, and yet I am still so bad at recognising it.

I begin to think of myself as a monster. Untrusting of my own memories and experiences, I fill the empty parts with fear and fantasy.

I feel that I am getting worse. Whenever I start to think seriously about premenstrual illness, I get distracted by *an evil to carry*. I become obsessed with female monsters, with how coming of age can be a metaphor for becoming evil.

—

At fifteen, a few months before my first period, I read Stephen King's *Carrie* (1974). For Carrie, a teenage misfit in an abusive home, the onset of puberty unleashes telekinetic powers. Her mother, who never taught Carrie about menstruation, calls it 'the Curse of Blood'.

Brian De Palma's 1976 film adaptation begins with slow-motion pans of young female bodies in a women's change room, scored by dreamy strings. Carrie is in the shower. She looks euphoric, almost orgasmic. Then she notices the blood. It's between her legs, dripping down her thighs. Euphoria ends. Panic sets in.

'Am I dying?' a terrified Carrie asks her gym teacher.

The mood echoes the famous shower scene in Alfred Hitchcock's 1960 film, *Psycho*: another tableau in which blissful solitude ends in horror. Here, the camera follows the blood as it runs down Carrie's legs and towards the drain. At the end of the scene, a light bulb flashes and breaks, and we hear two sharp notes, evocative of *Psycho*'s piercing, stabbing tones. But this time there is no shadow outside the shower. There is no external monster. The monster is inside the shower: inside Carrie.

The connection between blood and Carrie's telekinesis returns in the climax of the film. Carrie is crowned prom queen, but, once again, her joy is short-lived: when she's onstage accepting her title, her classmates douse her in pigs' blood. Humiliated, her powers grow forceful and frenzied, fuelled by rage. Her mother's voice ringing in her head, she annihilates everyone in the room—those who helped her and those who tormented her alike. She appears to be in a near-dissociative state, watching the world around her burn. Her rage is a product of her environment, but it's internal, too. Her display of anger seems half knowing revenge, half a loss of control.

In *Monster Theory*, Jeffrey Jerome Cohen posits that the creation of monsters is a way of policing behaviour within a society, ensuring that people do not defy cultural norms. What our culture views as a monstrosity shows us where the borders of polite society are, and what might happen if we dared to cross them. Betraying cultural expectations—be that by being too loud, too angry, too gay, too messy, or too different—can mean leaving the boundaries of what's culturally acceptable and entering the territory of the monster. It is to move beyond cultural reason, and 'risk attack by some monstrous border patrol or (worse) to become monstrous oneself'. Horror narratives then act as warnings: become too much, defy mainstream expectations, and risk becoming either a victim or a monster.

I think back to Carrie. To her mother, Carrie becomes monstrous the moment she gets her period. Becoming a woman is a transgression of childhood: a transgression of innocence. Yet to the audience, Carrie is monstrous only at the end of the film. Her real monstrosity is not her coming into adulthood, but her transgression of feminine ideals: her coming into rage.

There is more than one way to look at a monster. In Ovid's telling of the story of Medusa, the Gorgon was once a beautiful woman with lovely hair. She only became a monster after she was raped by Poseidon. Then her hair turned to snakes; direct eye contact turned men to stone. Put differently, her pain was so great that no one could bear to look at her. She was monstrous because she felt too much. Another of the Greek behemoths, Charybdis, was once a lusty, loud-mouthed woman. Zeus believed that she was stealing from him, so he chained her to the bottom of the ocean, where she would devour anything and everything in her path. She was cursed to become a voracious whirlpool. Her hunger could swell the tides. She wanted too much.

It's through these interpretations that I start to question my own biases and preconceptions: what is a monster, and who decides it is monstrous? Carrie's ability to transgress the cultural expectations of women as restrained—meek—is as enviable as it is fearsome. The horror is that in her revenge she hurts not only those who hurt her, but those who tried to help her, too. At the same time as I am horrified by her power, by her violence, I feel some sick admiration for her boundlessness, for the power she holds through her anger. Perhaps becoming a monster is not an inevitable ending, but a flash of power in an otherwise hopeless story.

Jess Zimmerman is an American writer whose work often explores gendered myths. In her book *Women and Other Monsters* Zimmerman is careful to remind us that most stories of monstrous women are stories told by men. From another viewpoint, these women are not monsters, but fleshy, angry, ambitious, desirous beings. Perhaps, were the stories written by these monstrous women, their narratives would feel less terrifying and more whole.

I see this same lack in other literature too: many of the resources I find about premenstrual illnesses are medical, scientific texts written—often by men—in disembodied and abstract ways. The illness is not lived in, but observed. I find the story told in these texts all the more distant, and at times useless, for it.

I think of the essay 'The Laugh of the Medusa', in which feminist critic Hélène Cixous writes, 'I wished that [women] would write . . . so that other women, other unacknowledged sovereigns, might exclaim: I, too, overflow; my desires have invented new desires, my body knows unheard-of songs.' Cixous writes of women who have learned to be ashamed of their strength, of their bodies and of their voices. She asks that women write not alongside these myths of monstrous women, but through and away from and despite them, that we write not because writing is good, but because, compared with these ancient stories of unspeakable horrors, it is new. There is immense possibility when, instead of writing reasonably, we write without reason.

'You only have to look at the Medusa straight on to see her. And she's not deadly. She's beautiful and she's laughing,' writes Cixous.

Perhaps a monster is just a body, or just a woman, and there are other stories we can tell.

10.

A supermoon blooms; it's 7 May 2020. The next day, Prime Minister Scott Morrison releases a three-step plan to liberate Australia from its cycles of lockdowns.

I slowly develop my own three-step plan to deal with this illness: first, I will remove my IUD to track a baseline. I want to give myself three months to notice my body without added hormones altering my cycle. I want to understand the ways in which this illness affects me and diagnose it properly. Then, if I truly am ill in the ways I believe myself to be, I will go on the pill—a newer one, one approved for treatment of PMDD. After three months, if the pill is not working, I will try an antidepressant. I have been forming this plan for months, but I am slow to act on it. Slow to do anything.

There is a secret fourth step that I do not talk about: hysterectomy.

The night before the first lockdown ends, Premier Daniel Andrews announces a road map to COVID-normal across Victoria. Visitors are allowed in the home: up to five per day. My phone dings with notifications from a million group chats as everyone tries to figure out who's seeing who. Three of our friends live together already. Eight people! In one house! It feels fantastical.

I'm as luteal as they come. I don't know it yet, but my period—and relief—won't arrive for ten days. My symptoms are starting earlier, and worsening. I lose track of what is *some of the time* and what is *all of the time.*

I cry reading a story about a Polish cow who escaped from a slaughterhouse. She broke a farmer's arm, ran through a fence and swam to safety. The farmers spent days trying to catch her, but whenever they got close, she dipped into the water and swam away. She made national headlines, was nicknamed the 'hero cow'. A Polish singer-turned-politician was so moved by her plight that he offered to buy her from the slaughterhouse so she could live out her days on his property in peace. I show Pavan the story, weeping, and ask him how we can love this cow and eat others. It's not like she wanted to live any more than the rest of them.

The next morning, in the kitchen, my housemate is butchering a quarter cow. He's laid it across the kitchen counter and is splitting it through the ribs with a butcher's knife. The meat is red and raw. The ribs are still ribs, the leg is still a leg. Pavan smiles at the housemate, says good morning, then turns me around and steers me down the hall.

'Let's go for a walk,' he says.

He takes me to Edinburgh Gardens and walks me around the footy oval. I feel frantic, like a caged animal, pacing lap after lap. I try to vent my frustration through words, but words embarrassingly turn to tears.

'I don't even care,' I say to Pavan, which is clearly not true. 'At least he's looking at the thing in the eye, butchering it himself, seeing it for what it is. He's not hiding behind words like *mince* or *steak* or *beef*.'

I go on my phone, try to find where the Polish cow is now. I discover that they managed to catch and tranquilise her. She woke in transit, freaked out and died from the stress. The ending feels hopelessly inevitable.

A notification pops up. In the group chat, our friends are texting plans for dinner.

I was thinking of making a vegetarian pie?

Like broccoli and mushroom?

Won't be vegan though

What's in it that isn't vegan?

Cream, butter, milk

Coz I could bring substitutes

I'll make my normal pie

The word *normal* makes me sting something abnormal. I don't understand *normal* anymore.

'I wish they'd just eat their dogs and be honest about it,' I tell Pavan, because it's confrontational enough to meet the anger dripping down my nose.

Pavan has never been an animal person. He's never had a dog or a cat. The first time I rode in his car, KFC boxes littered the floor, bones still inside. He pretended to be vegan to impress me, until somewhere along the way we both decided it was real. I ask him if it's hard, this thing that I'm making him do. I still think of it that way, like he doesn't have a choice.

Pavan holds my hand, takes me on another lap of the oval.

'It's not hard to be kind to you.'

We pace the oval until I'm lulled into a state of calm. He holds my hand until I can't remember where I end and he begins.

'Sorry I cry so much,' I tell him.

He shrugs, laughs.

'Whatever, dude,' he says. 'You're fine.'

Pavan makes a vegan stew to bring to dinner. We drive to North Melbourne with it. When our friends open the door, we hug. Overwhelmed, I burst into tears.

'Are those happy tears or sad tears?' one friend jokes. I'm not sure.

'I just can't believe I can see you again.'

We chat, hug again, laugh. I don't know how to make conversation anymore. Nothing has happened for the past month and a half. None of us have anything to talk about. We've all been pacing our bedrooms for six weeks straight. We place the food on the dining table, the pie the centrepiece.

'This pie is amazing,' someone says.

'Oh my god, you've killed it.'

'Thanks. It's the first time I've made it.'

I feel myself go berserk in place. I feel wild. The words *normal pie* and *first time* rollick through my head until I'm no longer normal.

I turn to Pavan, just to see if he hears it too, and he's serving himself a slice of normal pie.

He notices me notice him and there's no time to hide my reaction. I've got no poker face to begin with. I make an excuse, say I want to wash my hands, then cry stupid, frustrated tears in the bathroom. I stare myself down in the mirror, try to pull it together. I feel animal, out of control. Everything I want is right here—friends, freedom—and I'm miserable.

I imagine that I am a robot and attempt to return to some neutrality. Once I look normal enough, I go back downstairs, feign a smile, start filling my plate with sides. I don't look at Pavan again, don't trust myself to keep it together.

'The stew's great,' the friend who made the pie tells me.

'Thanks,' I smile. 'Pavan made it.'

She laughs and apologises: 'Sorry. I shouldn't assume just because you're the woman.'

Someone says something about the stew complementing the pie perfectly and it sounds like water in my ears. There's no point in being this upset. It doesn't make sense.

After dinner, a few of us go outside to smoke. I try to pour the water from my ears. I apologise to one of my friends, chalk it up to a bad vegan day.

'I get it,' they say. 'It's overwhelming, seeing everyone again.'

Pavan comes outside, too, but he doesn't look me in the eye. I think he's mad or maybe guilty. I'm reading too much into everything.

'We're talking about doing caps inside,' he says. 'Anyone want in?'

Everyone does. We ferry ourselves to the bedroom and split the caps between us.

My memory starts to fragment. We do drugs, dance, play spin the bottle. It feels feral, given the state of the world, but we all long to be feral. Suddenly, I'm away from the brink and moving towards solid ground.

I find Pavan on the stairs. He muffles out my apology with his own. The drugs have formed a blanket around me. I don't feel like crying.

'It's just a lot,' he says. 'It's been intense.'

'I know,' I say. 'I'm sorry.'

'I don't know how to handle it all the time.'

'I was so hurt,' I say.

'I know, I know,' he says. 'I think, for a moment, I just didn't want to care about hurting you. I wanted to be separate from you. But I don't want that anymore. I'm sorry.'

Downstairs, a man dressed as a Deliveroo driver is dropping off more drugs.

'It's never been this intense for me before,' Pavan says.

'You mean your past relationships?'

He nods and I feel myself still. It's the validation that I've been looking for: the problem is me. I am too much. Too intense. Too emotional. I am a monster. All of these things are true, objective facts, and the knowledge calms me, focuses me. I need to change.

'I'll get better,' I tell him. 'I promise.'

Our friends call out from downstairs. There's more MDMA, ketamine, all sorts.

In the early hours of the morning, Pavan and I crash in the spare room. He tells me with MDMA eyes that I've never looked so beautiful before. I tell him that I love him. It scares me, too, this intensity.

The next morning, I finally act on my plan. I make the appointment to get my IUD removed.

11.

'I'm taking it seriously this time,' I tell Pavan.

When I was first diagnosed at 22, I was told to track my symptoms. But I was lazy, and the hormonal IUD made my cycle irregular, so I did a poor job of it. Tracking my symptoms requires a kind of remembering that has always felt hazy to me. How can I begin to understand this illness when I don't even know my own body?

I make an appointment with my GP and tell her about my PMDD symptoms.

'I don't know much about PMDD,' my doctor admits. She looks it up on her computer, then suggests antidepressants.

I tell her about my plan: how I'll track a baseline without the IUD first, then go on the pill to see how my body responds. If that doesn't work, I will go on antidepressants, but I want it to be a last resort.

My doctor says removing the IUD is unlikely to make any difference. She suggests that I try all of these things at once and I baulk. There are too many independent variables. I want to understand my body and its spirals, to know what is wrong with me and what works to fix it.

I leave the appointment with a referral to get my IUD removed. I feel equal parts hope and defeat.

Later that night, I tell Pavan about the fourth stage, the hysterectomy, and he looks like he wants to cry. His reaction is more visceral than I'd expected. I feel surprised. Guilty. I don't even know if any of this will work. I'm just desperate for a road map out of here.

'Can't that wait?' he asks, as though I've already made the appointment.

Still, he doesn't push.

When my IUD was first inserted, my body became technologically altered. My period was no longer dictated by my biology alone. In 'A Cyborg Manifesto', Donna Haraway uses the metaphor of the cyborg to argue that to be human is no longer a wholly 'natural' state. 'By the late twentieth century, our time, a mythic time,' she writes, 'we are all chimeras, theorised and fabricated hybrids of machine and organism; in short, we are cyborgs.' She argues that, by the 1980s, the cyborgs of science fiction had become medical and lived realities. For Haraway, cyborgs are a pathway away from essentialist or rigid ways of thinking about bodily identities. She is critical of these binaries—of something either being 'natural' or not—and looks to the cyborg as a way of imagining more malleable ways of being; ways that don't give immutable boundaries to humans, animals, machines or even monsters.

Haraway first published her manifesto in 1985 in response to the socialist feminism of the time. She wanted to expand the movement's categories of women, class and patriarchy to create more fluid and intersectional ways of thinking and being—ways that could hold space for the shifting roles that race, sexuality, technology and culture play in shaping feminine and gendered experiences. Women are not one thing. Haraway poses the cyborg as an effective method for imagining these differences as both fluid and embodied.

I am interested in the way Haraway asks for gendered identities to transcend boundaries or borders—such as feminine expectations—by muddying the notion that those borders can exist at all. How can anyone expect a woman to represent Mother Nature, or the feminine divine, if she is technologically altered? To consider oneself entirely pure, or natural, is a fallacy that Haraway rejects in favour of more hybrid and connected ways of being.

Birth control—my IUD for example—is just one of many ways a person can be a cyborg. With an IUD inside me, I run against the narrative of Mother Nature, of woman-as-goddess, of the natural and divine woman. I am something mechanical, cyborg, hybrid—and a hybrid is a monster of its own. Personally, I have never been a fan of the goddess-woman trope. While I can understand why people find the notion of divine femininity liberating or empowering—it is a divergence from narratives of curses and lack, after all—I still find it hews too close to the dualistic narrative of woman as nature, man as human, that has existed throughout the history of Western philosophy. Instead of viewing a woman's power as something monstrous, it is seen as creative, divine and sacred. For me, this evokes images of fertile goddesses and balanced, moral women. The divine woman is a counter to female monstrosity, certainly, but it is a counter that exists too close to the dualism it tries to disrupt. I am a woman, I am an animal, I am nature, I am human—but all this should be too ordinary to be divine. By removing my IUD, I am becoming a little less cyborg and a little more human. I am getting closer to my 'natural' cycle, but to be more 'natural' is not to be more divine.

Before I read Haraway, all the cyborgs I could think of were men: Inspector Gadget, the Six Million Dollar Man, RoboCop. All good guys. The only female cyborg I was familiar with was Number Six from *Battlestar Galactica*. Number Six is a sexy vixen of a robot, disguised as a human. She's hot, thin, white. In the first episode, she wears a tight-fitting red dress, fucks a human, murders a baby and is instrumental in orchestrating the genocide of the human race. Here's yet another example of a woman transgressing the boundaries of femininity. Cyborgs lack feminine, motherly instincts—so become monsters instead.

There are other examples of female cyborgs, I am sure, but I cannot think of them. Instead, I think of Frankenstein's monster—a beast of fleshy parts, enlivened by technology. In Mary Shelley's *Frankenstein*, the monster is not a monster at all. They are not one singular thing, but an amalgamation of parts: rabbit, sow, woman, man. They are peaceful, vegetarian, intelligent. When Victor Frankenstein and the townspeople yell and shriek, they turn the creature into something to be rejected and feared, and so the creature stops seeking connection and becomes something fearsome instead. They—the creature—are a product of their environment; a product of a culture unable to see the sum of their parts as anything close to a whole.

'Though both are bound in the spiral dance, I would rather be a cyborg than a goddess,' writes Haraway. Despite my hope that it's the IUD, this cyborg part of me, that is making me crazy, I cannot help but agree. I am not removing my IUD to get closer to the divine. I don't expect my wild variability in mood to magically disappear, or that I'll suddenly find a spiritual connection with my period. Rather, it is an attempt to simplify things. I am hoping that I am removing one part of Frankenstein's monster—one unknowable variable—to better understand what I am like beneath it all. I hope I will be able to understand this illness rationally and diagnose it properly. But I also know that I can't solve for every variable. I cannot break my entire body down to its individual components and figure out what has gone wrong. I cannot account for my environment, either. I cannot know how I would feel were I not a caged animal, trapped indoors.

Pavan drives us to Doctors of Northcote on a Monday morning. I make him come inside with me: my birth control is his problem, too.

The doctor calls us in from the waiting room and we sit across the desk from her. She holds up a plastic model of a uterus to demonstrate the removal process. She places an IUD inside the uterus, then tugs it out through the plastic cervix by its string.

'See,' she says, putting the model down. 'Super quick and simple.'

'Wow,' says Pavan.

'Will it hurt?' I ask.

I can't see her expression behind her mask. She shrugs a little, says it doesn't hurt, but it's not exactly comfortable, either.

'So you're aware, you'll be fertile as soon as it's removed. There's no safe window.'

Pavan places a hand on my lower belly and says, 'Good, that's what we're hoping for.'

'He's kidding,' I say. 'We'll be safe.'

'We'll use abstinence,' Pavan says.

I ask her if I will bleed, and she says no, then pauses before admitting that there might be some spotting afterwards. I don't believe her. I am sure there will be blood.

'And your period will come back, of course. If it stopped with the IUD, that is.'

'It didn't stop entirely,' I say, 'but it was pretty infrequent. That's why I want to get it out—to see what my cycle is like without it.'

She hesitates before she responds. 'You know, I have a lot of patients who are concerned about not having their period for whatever reason—an IUD, the pill. They say it feels unnatural to miss it. I get that—but I don't think we were ever *really* supposed to have a regular period. Throughout most of our evolution, we've either been starving or pregnant. When you look at it that way, a regular period is a pretty modern thing.'

'Honestly, that makes me feel better about having a period,' I say. As much trouble as it has caused me, it sounds better than being starved and pregnant.

She leads me over to the examination bed and asks me to remove my pants, then turns away while I do so. The paper bedcover sticks to my arse. She hands me a disposable sheet for modesty. I'm amused by the pretence of it—as though she won't be opening me up and looking inside me within moments. Pavan stands behind me and rubs my shoulders.

I've never been embarrassed by doctors or pap smears. There's something about the clinical nature of it that distracts me from my own body. Sitting in a doctor's room, I feel less human and more object. My insecurities and modesties disappear under a doctor's gaze, my subjectivity wanes and I become a series of medical notes, or a case study. I think of our family dogs—how they always loved going to the vet, no matter how many thermometers were shoved up their arses.

The doctor picks up the speculum. I remember reading once that the design of the speculum has hardly changed in the two centuries since it was invented in the early 1800s. Around the same time, in 1816, a French physician called René Laennec invented the first stethoscope—then a trumpet-shaped device—to avoid the awkwardness of pressing his ears against his female patients' chests.

I'm doing it again—getting so distracted by the clinical process before me that I forget about my own body in the chair, my own legs spread wide in front of another human.

The doctor pumps some lube onto her gloves and warms it between her fingers before applying it to the speculum. 'Hopefully this won't be too cold,' she says.

It is cold.

She inserts the speculum and cranks it open, shines a small light inside me to help her find the IUD's string. Above me, Pavan is still rubbing my shoulders. He's all blue mask and big eyes.

'Aha,' says the doctor. 'Found it. Now get ready for a slight tugging sensation.'

Pavan squeezes my shoulders. 'Okay,' he says. 'Now push.'

I laugh, then gasp. I feel something like a tug, or a whoosh, like gravity has given way. She was right: this isn't pain, but something else, something unfamiliar, and maybe worse for it.

'All done,' she says.

'Woah,' I stutter. 'That was weird.'

'I know,' says the doctor. 'Our bodies aren't really used to things coming out like that.'

Quickly, my body stabilises and the discomfort fades, leaving only a shadow of the sensation.

'Do you want to see it?' the doctor asks. I do.

She shows me a little plastic tray with my IUD on it. It's the same as the one she used to demonstrate the procedure, only mine is flecked with brown. The string is muddy, crinkled. It looks lived-in.

'Gross,' I say.

She shrugs. 'Still looks pretty good to me.'

The morning after my IUD is taken out, I get my period in the shower. Or rather, my period falls out of me and slaps against the tiles in one monstrous glob. It's the scene from *Carrie*—prom night, not the opening shower scene—bright red, thick, more of it than I can imagine. I have to break the clots with my fingers to push them down the drain. Again, my body is acting abnormally, not doing what it's supposed to do. Afterwards, I feel the need to tell people—*Look what came out of me! Oh my god!*—like someone who has just taken a shit that is especially big, or long, or straight and intact, but no one wants to hear about it. I'm amazed by it, this personal body horror.

I bleed for eight days straight, like a purge.

In the kitchen, Pavan lets out a scream of pain.

'What happened?' I rush over to him. 'Did you cut yourself? Burn?'

'No, no,' he says. 'I had a cramp in my arse.'

I can't help but laugh. Earlier that day, at the chemist, a scorching pain had run through my guts, cervix, all the way down to my arse. It was seismic, electric. A cramp. I'd braced myself, breathed, and answered the chemist's questions with a neutral face. I hadn't even mentioned the pain.

'Imagine yelling because you had a cramp,' I say. Imagine! It sounds like a dream.

Little by little, the world opens up again. The bouldering gym near us reopens for members only, so we sign up. They're not doing rentals, so Pavan helps me pick out a pair of climbing shoes to buy. They're painfully tight.

'They're meant to be,' says the sales assistant. 'Have you worn uncomfortable shoes before?'

I want to tell him that I spent my teen years sprinting up and down the hill from Macleod station in platform heels, trying to get home before my parents did. I want to tell him that I am a woman, and I know the difference between discomfort and pain. Instead, I try the too-tight shoes on again and say they're too tight, again. He doesn't believe me—I'm not a very good climber, after all—but I buy the shoes I want anyway. They're uncomfortably tight, but not painfully so. At the end of our first session, my heels are rubbed raw and blistered.

Within weeks, I learn that my doctor is right. Removing the IUD makes little to no difference; my moods swing low all the same. The only change is that my cycle becomes more regular, my tides more predictable.

I begin to see monsters as a way of coping with this illness.

'The horizon where the monsters dwell might well be imagined as the visible edge of the hermeneutic circle itself,' writes Jeffrey Jerome Cohen in *Monster Theory*. 'The monstrous offers an escape from its hermetic path, an invitation to explore new spirals, new and interconnected methods of perceiving the world.'

Alone in my room, slowly spiralling inwards, I imagine what it would be like to spiral out instead. Eventually, an inward spiral runs out of room. Its turns grow small; its walls draw closer and closer. It closes in on itself. I want to make room for myself, to push back against this story I am carving myself. I want to push outwards into infinite nothing. I want to do the wrong thing.

I imagine what it would be like to make my pain, my discomfort, someone else's problem. To say, *I am in pain, look at me.* I still feel—surprisingly strongly—that this act would be a monstrous one and that, perhaps, I am monstrous for even thinking it. 'Through the body of a monster,' Cohen writes, 'fantasies of aggression, domination, and inversion are allowed safe expression.' At the same time as I fear becoming these monsters, I envy them. They are a safety net, a fantasy. I want to be them: unrestrained, uninhibited. It's this fear-desire that keeps me circling myth and magic, wondering what it means to be a monster and which impulses, if I allowed myself, I might act on.

My sense of self starts to fracture, and I lose track of the who's-who of it all. I no longer know which version of myself—my ill-self or my well-self—indulges in violent fantasies: fantasies of screaming, ripping my clothes off, punching the walls, yelling at Pavan, my housemates, my boss. There are days when I am sure—certain—that it is my ill-self who harbours these fantasies. Surely, she is the one with the monstrous desires. But then comes the doubt. When I am unwell, I fear myself. I am so terrified of what I *might* do that I hardly do anything at all. When I speak out a little, I fear I've gone too far. More likely, it is my well-self who wants to be monstrous: who wants it to be that simple and revelatory. If I were to spiral outwards, not in, perhaps I could feel what it's like to truly transgress this body. Perhaps I could escape this discomfort, and instead indulge purely in desire, emotion, instinct.

12.

In 1980, the same year that Sandie Craddock killed her co-worker, Christine English sat in her car, stared down her lover and stepped hard on the accelerator. She pinned her boyfriend, Barry, between her car and a lamp post. It was two weeks before Christmas. Unlike Sandie, Christine had no prior convictions. No history of violence, no manic outbursts. She hadn't eaten in nine hours.

Later, in court, Katharina Dalton, the expert witness in Sandie Craddock's trial, would testify that 'in cases of premenstrual tension sufferers, lack of food causes an aggressive, impatient condition through adrenalin being released into the blood leading to increased irritability and tension'. Hunger becomes outsized. Rage becomes outsized.

I'm drawn to the ways in which women's violence is written as the manifestation of some internal lack: hunger, fatigue. In *Diseases of Women*, the first record of hysteria, Hippocrates wrote that 'if the woman does not have intercourse with her husband, and her belly is emptier at this time because of some pain, then the womb displaces itself'. A lack in the stomach, a lack in the womb.

'Outsize hunger is the province of the monster, and for women, all hunger is outsize,' writes Jess Zimmerman in her book *Women and Other Monsters*. For Zimmerman, the ancient behemoths represent a patriarchal fear. Consume too much, want too much, feel too much, and become a monster. She writes of Charybdis, that stormy sea monster who, alongside her sister Scylla, devoured and destroyed any ship that tried to pass. She was cursed to become a monster, cursed to consume.

The horror I enjoy most is that of the horrific woman. *Jennifer's Body*, *Carrie*, *Raw*. In most of these stories, the women devour something disgusting: raw chicken, human flesh. In most of these stories, the women kill men.

Those close to Christine described her relationship with Barry as tumultuous. Christine was divorced, with two kids. Barry had a wife. He was unemployed, drank a lot. Some days, when Barry had drunk more than usual, which was not unusual, he would hit her. He always apologised afterwards. He always promised to reform.

On the morning before Christine killed Barry, he cancelled their dinner plans, telling her he had a date with another woman. She yelled; he got violent. He left for the pub. Christine tracked him down, confronted him again. She followed him out of the bar, made him get in her car and drove him all around town looking for this other woman. When that failed, they went to another pub, drank more, fought again. She yelled; he hit. When Barry asked Christine to drive him home, she refused. More fighting, more violence. Spiralling.

'I hate you and I never want to see you again,' Barry yelled.

Christine drove off. Then, on the way home, she had a change of heart. She turned around, looking to pick Barry up and make peace. When she found him, he flashed a backwards V-sign at her. *Up yours.* That's when she smashed him against a lamp post.

Christine, 'hysterical but clear-headed', an implausible duality, was taken to the local police station. On release the next morning, at 5 a.m., she began to menstruate.

Barry died in hospital two weeks later.

Like Sandie, Christine pleaded guilty to manslaughter with reduced responsibility. She, too, suffered from premenstrual tension.

'I do not think it would serve any purpose to send you to prison,' the Judge told Christine. She received twelve months' probation with a driving ban.

After Christine's release, Barry's widow spoke to reporters. 'Other women have to live with and control premenstrual stress and tension. It seems wrong that women can now use this as an excuse for anything,' she said.

When I read Christine's story, she strikes me less as a woman struggling with menstrual illness, and more as a woman driven mad by her environment. She was a victim of domestic violence. Unlike Sandie, Christine had no prior record, no history of violent outbursts, no constellations of bad behaviour. It wasn't until that day with Barry that her anger finally became outsized and she lashed out.

I start to wonder if what I feel during my luteal phase is justified rage at an unfair world, and the rest of the time I am just numb enough to tolerate the unfairness around me. Or perhaps I am not very resilient. I've never hurt anyone, never run anyone down with my car. Yet Pavan is no Barry. If I were to find myself in Christine's circumstances, were I to be mocked and ridiculed and beaten, I can't say with any certainty that I wouldn't.

In Switzerland, in 1459, Catherine Simon of Andermatt confessed to having transformed into a wolf with the aid of herbal witchcraft. This is the earliest record I could find of a human facing trial for transforming into a wolf. While in her wolf form, she claimed to have run alongside the devil and caused an avalanche. She confessed to other crimes, too: inflicting illness, killing livestock, attempting murder, more avalanches. Catherine struck such horror in her community that her executioner was asked to 'divide her into two pieces, of which one shall be her head and the other her body, which shall be so completely severed that a cartwheel can be rolled between them'. Afterwards, her severed remains were burnt, then, as though that were not enough to kill her, her ashes were cast into a river.

In the 1980s, premenstrual dysphoric disorder was a controversial potential addition to the *Diagnostic and Statistical Manual of Mental Disorders* (DSM). Many psychiatrists pushed back against the inclusion of PMDD as a psychiatric illness for fear that it would further stigmatise a normal part of menstruation. I think of female werewolves, how they ask their doctors, the school nurse, *What is wrong with me?* and are told, *This is normal.*

Over the course of 1986, the debate over PMDD took place across oversight bodies, in closed-door discussions, at protests, in newspapers and public debates. When the DSM-III-R was published in 1987, PMDD was ultimately excluded as an official disorder. Instead, it was mentioned under the name *late luteal phase dysphoric disorder*, or LLPDD: a proposed disorder in need of further research. For the first time, a formal diagnostic procedure was drafted. As work began on the DSM-IV, organisers knew that the inclusion or exclusion of menstrual illness within the diagnostic manual would remain contentious. Hysteria had only been removed from the manual in 1980, and the profession was still trying to shake off its legacy. Some doctors worried that PMDD was simply a new name for a long history of misogyny. They feared the kind of sexism that my own mother faced in the workforce in the 1980s: that women would be dismissed as unreliable, untrustworthy and incapable during *that time of the month*.

Their fears were understandable. In the early twentieth century, Freud's notion of hysteria as a 'psychological neurosis' dominated the medical and psychotherapeutic landscape. The myth of the hysteric was used to diminish and stigmatise women, and as an argument against women's advancement and suffragette movements. The connective tissue between hysterical neurosis and premenstrual illness is strong. In 1931, gynaecologist Robert Frank reconnected hysteria's psychological neurosis to a hormonal cause, making the case that these nervous conditions, once thought to be brought on by a displaced womb, an empty stomach, or even a missing penis, were actually brought on by the menstrual cycle. Frank first described the symptoms of premenstrual dysphoric disorder under the name *premenstrual tension*. When I read the word *tension*, I have to admit that it feels apt—in the luteal phase I do feel as though I am wound too tight and on the edge of snapping. Simply by being unwell in the way that I am, I feel that I, too, am legitimising some sexist, irrational, uncontrollable trope.

Frank believed that premenstrual tension was due to an excess of oestrogen, causing fluid retention before menses. The symptoms he described included fatigue, attacks of pain, irritability, headaches, swollen faces, hands or feet, asthma, epileptic seizures and 'foolish actions'. Alongside bed rest, Frank prescribed dehydration methods to treat premenstrual tension: coffee or tea diuretics, designed to expel excess oestrogen from the body through piss and sweat.

Katharina Dalton later expanded on Frank's work with her partner Raymond Greene, renaming premenstrual tension as *premenstrual syndrome*, or *PMS*, in 1953. While training as a general practitioner, Dalton had observed that her migraines seemed to amplify at certain times of the month, and disappear at others. In response, she began tracking the symptoms of her female patients in line with their menstrual cycles. She drew connections between the stages of their menstrual cycles—ovulation, luteal, menses—and their moods. Though she would never prove it, she believed that some women had hormonal imbalances, leading to abnormal, uncontrolled mood swings, or PMS. Despite her lack of biological proof, her work was instrumental to the debate around PMS and PMDD.

Many of the symptoms of PMDD are the same traits that women are raised to quell within themselves: anger, irritation, feeling out of control. Nada Stotland, a psychiatrist who would later become president of the American Psychiatric Association, was sceptical about PMDD's inclusion within the DSM. She asked that her fellow committee members think carefully about gender roles before turning one gender's humanity into an illness. Her concerns were fair: without considering the ways in which women had been raised and conditioned to view themselves, the committee risked turning a woman's regular anger, stress and irritation into a disease.

'Women are often paid less, put in subordinate positions, occasionally beaten up at home, and nowadays have to earn a significant portion of the family income and be responsible for the family home, where they do the lion's share of the work—and they're still asked not to be angry, and always to be in control,' Stotland said in an interview with journalist Karen Houppert. 'So, all of those things don't mean there's no such thing as PMDD, but that it's very hard to establish hormones as the cause of these feelings.'

I try to remember that two things can be true. Hormones can be debilitating, and a culture can be debilitating, too. Not every person who was raised as a woman, who lives a stressful life, or who experiences gendered injustice, develops premenstrual symptoms. There are many people who believe in premenstrual syndrome, who work, who care for large families, who do most of the household work, who are overrun and overstressed, and yet do not experience premenstrual stress, tension, dysphoria. Similarly, not every person who does experience premenstrual stress is female—trans men and nonbinary people have been diagnosed with it, too, despite often rejecting the gendered roles illnesses like PMDD are said to embody. Regardless of these complications, our culture is structured in such a way that an illness must be named before it can be treated. By avoiding naming PMDD as an illness, we limit the avenues available for those who cannot manage their anger—who cannot function—to seek help.

Premenstrual dysphoric disorder was finally included as a psychiatric illness in the DSM-V in 2013. For the first time, women could seek formal diagnosis and treatment. Doctors could apply for grants to study PMDD, research could be directed towards finding a cure, medicine, a biological cause. I, only two years later, could be diagnosed with it. It is because of this inclusion—and diagnosis—that I can see a psychologist, seek different treatments. When I hear that medicine is decades behind what it could be when it comes to understanding premenstrual illness, I think the story of the DSM gets part way to why. There has been so much debate—so much sexism, taboo and stigma—that it feels impossible to honestly understand this illness. All those years of discussion were years of missed research and missed funding.

I understand the concerns around naming this thing. I think they are well founded, even. I can see the sexism in reducing a person to their biology—to their hormonal influences. Yet at the same time, I think it's naive to view us as *other* than our hormones, our biology. Perhaps the sexism stems from the ways in which we view women as susceptible to hormones, and men as exempt.

I also understand that, while this codification represents progress, there is still much to be wary of. The diagnostic criteria for PMDD are strict, yet also broad. A woman who fights with her boyfriend over the dishes each month could be deemed irritable and conflict-seeking. By categorising PMDD as a mental disorder, we risk turning women's anger into a pathology. Simultaneously, there was very little biological evidence for the existence of PMDD at the time of its inclusion. There were no abnormal levels of hormones, no traceable causes. It seemed likely, given the evidence, that women could be hurt by this diagnosis. That they could experience the normal ebbs and flows of their menstrual cycle, and be deemed crazy for it, and believe themselves to be crazy, too. For centuries, hysteria was wielded as a tool to write off women's distress—the distress that made men uncomfortable—and turn it into a pathology. The removal of this diagnosis marked a change in the way medical institutions viewed women: as somehow weaker, more biologically fallible, vulnerable to shifts in tide or moon. How harmful, it seems, to let this same Cartesian dualism slip through under a new name.

I understand all these fears—I do. There are days when I feel like a sexist cliché: unable to work due to *women's issues*. Just as a placebo can make an illness better, the labelling of something as an illness can also make it worse. Menstruation is already loaded with so much stigma. I feel the burden of my own biases against myself. When I am premenstrual, I don't trust my feelings. I don't trust myself to speak out and be reasonable. Undeniably, this makes my symptoms worse.

Yet alongside medicine's history of pathologising women runs a parallel history of bias: of not listening to women and not taking their pain seriously. This can be seen in the way women's pain is dismissed in emergency rooms, in how few medical experiments include women.

Even crash-test dummies are almost exclusively modelled after men. Male height, male build, male shape. Tests might include a shrunken-down male dummy in lieu of a female one, as though to be a woman is to be a smaller man. I'm unsurprised when I learn that women are more likely to suffer from whiplash than men.

Menstrual illness is so often misunderstood, misdiagnosed or mythologised because we still know so little about illnesses that affect women more than men. Science is still playing catch-up. While excluding PMDD from the DSM would perhaps be a step away from the tendency to pathologise women, I'm unsure if it would get us anywhere closer to listening to them. One hundred years ago, my symptoms would have fit under the cluster of hysteria: I would have been treated with vibrators and baths instead of pills. Perhaps the pain I feel bends and shapes itself to the name I am able to give it, but underneath all that remains something altogether unnameable: the experience itself.

More than a quarter of women who are diagnosed with PMDD are first misdiagnosed with a different psychiatric disorder. In my experience, the diagnostic process has always been haphazard: a set of check boxes medical specialists use to push me through the system. To make a referral. To give a prescription. My medical records have scattergun markings of generalised anxiety, mild depression, disordered eating—no diagnosis ever quite fitting the exact criteria of its DSM listing.

One common misdiagnosis for people with PMDD is bipolar disorder. Like PMDD, the exact causes for bipolar disorder are unknown; perhaps it's a combination of genetic, environmental and social factors all swirling together, making someone more likely to fall into the cycles of mania and depression that are characteristic of bipolar.

As I begin to track my cycle without an IUD, I become increasingly sure that the diagnosis of PMDD is the right one. I also become aware of the many adjacent categories my illness could have fallen into instead, were my symptoms looked at through a slightly different lens. I am thankful that I was never misdiagnosed with bipolar, that I didn't spiral down a different rabbit hole, seeking even more help that never quite worked. While my body cycles through lows, it doesn't quite express the highs that most doctors look for when diagnosing bipolar. PMDD seems a closer fit. Yet reading through my journals, trying to remember how this illness absorbs my body, I see that the contrast between my two selves contains a mania of its own. My well-self reads as more deranged than my ill-self. How strange, to want to die one day, and to believe that yoga could cure me the next.

I think back to the doctor at the bulk-billing clinic, how a little term in a big book was enough for him to get me out of his office within half an hour. Had he stumbled across any other term—*bipolar, borderline, hysteria*—he may have diagnosed me under the umbrella of those symptoms instead.

I search through my medical records, looking for what he wrote about me, how, with the little information he had, he arrived at this particular diagnosis, how it happened to feel right. In his appointment notes, he writes that I have 'a child-like affect'. When I read it, I can't help but roll my eyes.

How lucky I would have to be, I think, *for such a happenstance diagnosis to be right.*

Throughout *In the Dream House*, author and critic Carmen Maria Machado writes about domestic violence in lesbian relationships and the confounding societal response. Women, it is generally believed, are victims, not abusers. There's both sexism and homophobia in our unwillingness to see women as perpetrators. Throughout her memoir, she retells the historic story of a woman named Alice, who killed her lover, Freda, in a fit of jealous rage.

'I resolved to kill Freda because I loved her so much that I wanted her to die loving me,' Alice wrote in a statement. To me, she sounds like every cliché of domestic violence. But to a jury in the nineteenth century—to a jury who could not fathom a woman's love for another woman, who could not reckon with the reality that women can love, and be jealous, and be angry, and be violent—she sounded like a madwoman. Alice was sentenced to life in an insane asylum.

When a woman commits a crime, she transgresses the expectations of a meek femininity. She is driven by masculine, violent impulses, and is thus unfathomable. When a suspect doesn't match the profile, it's easier, perhaps, to deem her insane.

For their respective juries, Sandie Craddock and Christine English offered two possible narratives: they were monstrous women, or they were madwomen. In a culture that views women as meek, kind and motherly, it was easier to imagine two women driven mad by the very nature of their biology than to imagine the fullness of their desire and rage.

In the years following Sandie and Christine's trials, legal publications bloomed with analysis of 'the PMS defence'. On one side of the debate was the request that women who suffer from premenstrual illnesses be treated with compassion, that their circumstances be taken into account. On the other side, lawyers argued that the diagnostic criteria for premenstrual illnesses were too broad, that the evidence was sketchy at best, that women should not be patronised and victimised, that they should be considered agents of their crimes. Some lawyers feared that allowing for a premenstrual defence would bring about the rebirth of Freudian hysteria, where upset women were deemed in need of a good fuck, or dismissed as irrational due to *that time of the month.*

Is a woman who kills a monster or madwoman? I no longer find the binaries useful.

In today's courts, Christine English would have more likely relied on a battered woman defence than one of premenstrual illness. Battered woman syndrome emerged as a legal defence in the 1990s in response to a series of crimes in which abused women murdered their abusive husbands. Unlike a plea of self-defence, the battered woman defence argues that the victim was acting in defence against cumulative acts of abuse, rather than one singular provoking incident. In the United Kingdom, where Christine and Sandie were tried, battered woman syndrome is not considered a whole defence. Rather, like the premenstrual defence, it can go some of the way towards establishing the reduced culpability of the accused.

Yet, in the early 1980s, some jurors were more likely to view Christine as responsible for Barry's violence than they were to view her as responsible for her menstrual rage. As one lawyer wrote in the footnotes of his case notes: 'English, like any woman, is responsible for choosing a violent alcoholic married man as her lover and remaining with him . . . Her excuse is limited to premenstrual "spleen and vapours".'

I find it neither a stretch nor a leap to imagine that Christine felt at least partly responsible for the violence she experienced at the hands of her boyfriend. I also find it no stretch of the imagination to believe that she felt maddened by this responsibility. I find her rage explicable, even rational, if outsized. I take a fictive leap and imagine that, at the police station, after her arrest, she, too, was looking for any way to rationalise her own responsibility and guilt for Barry Kitson's death. I imagine her leaving the police station, feeling a rush of red, and looking to blame her own animal body for her violent anger.

13.

The Friday after my IUD removal is Pavan's birthday. We're meeting friends in Royal Park. He'd spent the evening before on his phone, frantic about who might be there, who might be late. Numbers are still a delicate balance.

When he sees how I am dressed the next morning, he makes a face.

'Are you really wearing that?' he asks.

'It's comfortable.' I'm wearing the loosest clothing I own.

'Don't wear that,' he says. 'There will be photos, you know.'

'So?'

'I don't want you to regret it.'

I can't tell whether he's being mean or stupid. My body tightens, ready to argue.

'Please,' he says.

I make a face, like he's being ridiculous, but sullenly agree to change.

It's his birthday, after all.

I don't tell him that I don't want to change because I feel wrong in my body. My clothes are too tight, and I can't tell whether it's the lockdown weight or my own thoughts that make me feel that way.

I change into black jeans and a black shirt. I can tell he's unsatisfied with my choice, but he doesn't ask again.

At the park, Pavan drops down on one knee and holds out a thin silver ring. We don't say anything, just hug. Our friends cheer, take photos. We pop a bottle of champagne and the foam goes everywhere.

We drop acid and the ground melts and spirals.

I keep looping through the same thoughts, approaching them from different angles. How funny it is that Pavan proposed to me. How sweet to plan it for his birthday. On one spiral, I can't stop laughing at the silliness of it all. On another, the gesture is too much, too serious, too real. I remember a fact from somewhere: how marriage makes men happier, and women sadder. I'd never dreamed of getting married, never fantasised about my own wedding. I think that I like it better this way, getting married when it feels impulsive and dangerous, rather than waiting for it to become an expected, sensible thing.

Day turns to night, and ten of us move back to a friend's house—the new limit, per government guidelines. Pavan and I lie with the friend on her bed. He'd once had a crush on her, when they were at uni. Over the summer, he told me about the sudden intensity of his feelings back then. He'd drunkenly pulled her aside at a party and told her that he loved her. She'd turned him down.

She asks if she can plan our wedding for us, says that she's always loved weddings.

I shrug: sure, if she wants to. From her wall, Harry Styles stares down at us. I think that Pavan's is a boy-band type of love: sweet, charming, cool, unthreatening, a little bit goofy.

'How funny,' says the friend, 'to think that it could have been me.'

I think I should feel jealous, but I just feel guilty. Here is a boy who wants to marry me—supposed to be some little girl's dream—and I can hardly take it seriously at all.

Time moves slowly: minutes pass like hours. One friend has a bad time, and it starts to freak everyone out. I become more aware than ever of how each of us is pulling and orbiting around the others.

'Is he okay?' another friend asks. She looks worried. I'm worried, too. He's walking stiffly, like a robot, like the whole world might implode if he relaxes his face. It's terrifying.

'I think the more that we're okay, the more he'll be okay.'

It's a lucky guess. A few of us take turns sitting with him, and eventually the real world breaks through. He comes to, shakes his head, asks for an ibuprofen and a lasagne.

'I think acid and proposals are a bad combo,' I tell Pavan once I no longer see the world in swirls. 'I haven't been able to stop thinking about it.'

'Oh yeah,' Pavan says. 'I forgot that happened today. Wild.'

I'm embarrassed. I've spent the whole day thinking about marriage, alone.

Then Pavan says: 'Holy shit, we're getting married.'

And it sounds so joyfully simple.

I cannot think of a good, rational reason to get married. Not so long ago, marriage represented social certainty, an exchange of goods, an enhanced political reputation, a guarantee that this baby is yours. Pavan and I will receive no tax benefits from getting married. There will be no exchange of goods. Relations between countries will not improve due to our union. If we were to have a baby—a big if—our marriage would not be the most reliable test of genetic lineage available to us.

In *Trick Mirror*, Jia Tolentino writes of the historical inequality of marriage: 'There is still a dramatic mismatch between the cultural script around marriage, in which a man grudgingly acquiesces to a woman salivating for a diamond, and the reality of marriage, in which men's lives often get better, and women's lives often get worse.' I worry that I am laying traps for myself. I don't want a diamond, I don't fantasise about my wedding, but that does not make me any less foolish. In the 1970s, it was the women who took on more traditional gender roles—who were married, who stayed home and cared for kids—who reported more severe premenstrual symptoms. I am sure that this reflects a cultural malaise, a frustration with the oppressive culture of the times. I have more options than these women. I am not expected to be any one thing. I wonder if I am deluding myself into thinking that this is a good idea simply because I am so terribly bored.

I do not know who Pavan will be in ten years. I do not know who I will be. When I think of marriage rationally, I can only think of it as a mistake. But I am trying not to think rationally. The year is already drawing out. We have seen pandemic, fires, floods. I am looking for anything like hope. Of all the bad things in the world, divorce seems almost manageable. Even if it ends, what a joy to have started.

A few days later, Pavan and I visit my parents for lunch.

While Dad's upstairs, I blurt out that we're getting married. Mum looks horrified. Pavan does, too. He's only met my parents a handful of times in the months we've been dating, and mostly via Zoom. He'd thought we'd ease them into this. When my dad comes down, he sees our faces and asks what happened. I deliver the news again, apologetic this time.

'Congratulations,' he says. 'Okay.'

By the time we leave, my mum is near tears.

'I'm sorry, Pavan,' she says. 'This isn't about you. I'm sure you're great. I'm just really invested in her happiness.'

In the car, Pavan and I exchange awkward glances.

'I shouldn't have said it like that, should I?' I say.

'Probably not.'

His parents live ten minutes from mine, so we decide to bite the bullet and do the double whammy.

'Hey, Mum,' Pavan says when we get inside. 'We're getting married.'

His mum waves a hand like it's no big deal, says, 'Good, you should settle down.'

—

I google *cheapest marriage celebrants in Melbourne* and come up with a woman named Julie, who charges less than the Melbourne Town Hall. There aren't many places we're legally allowed to visit, so we arrange to meet at a McDonald's in Richmond. We find her in a booth, then order coffees from the McCafé.

'You know,' she says, 'I specialise in multicultural weddings.'

She asks us how we found her, and I make up a lie about reading good reviews. To be honest, I haven't even looked at her reviews.

'So, why are you getting married?'

I say, 'Because we love each other,' because it sounds better than, 'Because we can.'

She asks us what we do for work, and we tell her that we're both writers: him for TV, me in a more abstract sense. Pavan name-drops the TV show he writes for, because it's been running for 40 years and tends to be a hit with a certain demographic, but Julie just makes a face and says that she was never a fan. She says she's a writer, too, but in a way that's designed to upsell us to a more expensive wedding package in which she will tell our love story for us.

'We really just want the legal-only package,' we say.

She asks us if we have shared views on religion, kids. We tell her that we don't really think about either.

I can tell that we're answering the questions all wrong, being too nonchalant. She seems put off that we don't have any grand visions of marriage, that we don't seem particularly romantic about it. I remember hearing something about marriage celebrants not being allowed to perform a ceremony if they believe that the institution of marriage is being made a mockery of, so I try to toe the line.

'When you know, you know,' I tell her, and that seems to do the trick. It's a slow year for weddings. She's not about to get picky.

'I can't believe we're actually doing it,' I say on the drive home.

'I kind of love Julie,' Pavan says.

I realise that the reason I want to marry Pavan is because he is telling himself the same story as I am telling myself. It's not settling down, it's not throwing away a future, it's not kids and religion and sacrifice. Despite having just said *when you know, you know*, I honestly believe most people don't know, even when they know. The kind of knowing I have with Pavan is not that this is my person, this is the so-called 'it', but rather that we're writing the same story together, and I trust his version of our world. When he says *marriage*, he means the same thing I do. We have the same language for this.

'Are we doing this as a joke, or for real?' I ask later that night, during a moment of uncertainty.

He shrugs, tells me that two things can be true.

14.

In the last week of June, one of my housemates says he's moving out—the one who butchers cows on the kitchen counter. I'm secretly thrilled.

I propose to the other housemates the idea of Pavan moving in, and they agree.

'He's here all the time anyway,' they say, and it sounds like a good thing.

We'll have two rooms now: a bedroom and a study.

I've been tracking my cycle for two months. The week before he moves in is the week before my period. I'm terrified that I will blow up our cohabitation before it even starts.

On an ABC podcast, Laura Murphy described her PMDD in terms of grief.

Each month, in the week or so before her period, she would sleep for twelve to thirteen hours, wake up, eat, then return to bed for another nap. She was unable to work. She would become despondent, staring at walls, the ceiling, into space. When questioned by her partner, she would become weepy.

'It's just such a bizarre experience,' she said. 'It felt like going through a bereavement every month, like my chest would just hurt with pain and suffering, and you'd sob and sob and sob and you'd know deep down that it wasn't because of anything, if that makes sense. But you just felt so much pain that you couldn't stop it.'

Of all the descriptions I have heard of PMDD—of monsters, of losing control, of anger and irritation—this one feels closest to the truth. I do not know how I can hold so much inside me.

For the seventeen years before she was diagnosed, Laura couldn't keep a job, and was barely functional for up to twelve days before her period. After undergoing a procedure to induce surgical menopause, she was able to slowly pull her life back together. She now works for the International Association for Premenstrual Disorders (IAPMD), a support and advocacy network for people with PMDD. She has a job, a house, three cats—all small impossibilities when her health was at its worst.

Two months into tracking a baseline, and my pattern becomes as predictable as a lunar calendar. For a week and a half before my period, I am miserable. I sleep for hours; when awake, I stare at the ceiling. I feel overwhelmed and out of control, like all this feeling is going to force its way out of me somehow. I can't work, can't think, can't do anything. I lie on the ground next to my computer, begging myself to just answer an email, upload a fact sheet, do something. I don't understand why I can't—why I won't. I focus instead on the tasks that I can write up in my end-of-day report. It's busywork. Then my period comes and my mood lifts. I come to my senses. I spend the week catching up on everything I let slip the week before. I feel fuelled, motivated. I want to make things right again.

I'm replaying the same routine over and over: dropping too many balls, then scrambling to pick them all up again.

When I look at my calendar of moods, I see all this and more. Yet what surprises me the most are not the sad days, but the happy ones. For two and a half weeks after my period begins, I am content—happy, even. I had not expected to find myself happy. I don't know how to hold these two things as true: I am both well and unwell.

In *Illness as Metaphor*, Susan Sontag writes, 'Illness is the night-side of life . . . Everyone is born with dual citizenship, in the kingdom of the well and the kingdom of the sick.' Many people who experience mental illness describe a severing of selves, and I feel this severing most clearly when I see my good days for what they are. The ill-self and the well-self: I imagine myself threading these identities together, making something solid from the parts of the whole.

In July, Pavan moves in. We move the bed to the new room—the upstairs room—and turn my room into a study. We spend an afternoon arranging the desks. It feels like a circuit breaker. Perhaps, if I am no longer pacing circles between my desk and my bed, I will be happier.

Still, it's not enough. I'm unable to do anything outside of work. I try to make time for creative projects. I submit pieces to a couple of publications, ask my friends if they want to start a zine. Only one friend shares her work. Her poem consists of the words *DON'T SPIRAL* written over and over, forming loops across the page.

I start to dread walks with friends. I don't want to leave the house, don't want to make conversation. No one has anything to say, anyway. Everyone fixates on the smallest things: a missed call, a bad look, a misstep, sends tremors through the friendship group. I, too, am fixating on the small stuff. On a walk, a friend complains about her housemate, and I find myself hating the housemate, too. All this boredom, all this anger, is easy to misplace.

Later, at Fitzroy Coles, Pavan asks me which pasta I'd prefer, and I spend a lifetime looking at the packages. I feel like I can't read them, though that's not quite true. The words are there, but they are strange and obtuse. I stare at the rows and rows of brightly coloured boxes, struck by each minuscule variation.

'What does this mean?' I say, pointing to a star on one of the packages that says *Made from immune-boosting ingredients.*

'It's just marketing,' says Pavan, which doesn't quite answer my question.

For the first time, I feel as though I'm seeing the supermarket for what it really is: an absurd landscape filled with an overwhelming array of choices. I stare and stare at the packages, trying to decipher which ones are vegan.

'You want that?' Pavan says when he notices me holding a packet of vegan jelly.

'I don't know,' I answer honestly. 'I don't want anything.'

Pavan rolls me through the aisles.

'Garlic,' I tell him, a memory I don't know what to do with.

'Good catch,' he says and lets me wait by the trolley as he runs to grab some.

Later that night, I reassociate and am turned sideways by the flood of sadness, terror and dread that follows. I go to a friend's house out of fear that I've worn Pavan thin. There's only so long I can ask one person to carry this with me. I sit on the friend's couch, ask her to carry it instead. I describe the experience in the supermarket, and she understands.

'It's anxiety,' she says. 'Your body is so prepped for fight-or-flight that normal things don't matter anymore. Your body is trying to absorb too much at once. The filters are off. What does your brain care about garlic when you could die at any moment?'

15.

Pavan and I try to make a habit of climbing. My head starts buzzing as soon as we enter the gym. Pavan, ahead of me, laces up his climbing shoes and pulls the chalk from his bag.

'Want to warm up?' he asks.

I tell him I'll be there in a second. I fold myself into one of the blue pleather couches. My head feels empty, catastrophically so. I sit on the couch and note what I can see: red holds on the wall, a languid greyhound snoozing beside a potted palm, bottles of liquid chalk on the coffee table, a woman effortlessly swinging up a green route, polished concrete floors. Then, what I can hear: laughter, the slap of feet against crash mats, mellow beats through the gym's speakers, Pavan saying: 'Hey, you're scaring me.'

'Oh, sorry,' I say with a start. It's like I'm talking through anaesthesia. 'I was doing that exercise where you list things. It's supposed to calm you down.'

'Do we need to leave?' He sounds frustrated. This is not the first time I've ruined bouldering.

'No,' I say. I can tell it's freaking him out, my lack of explanation, but I can't bring myself to say more. 'I'll take a walk,' I say instead.

I sit outside near the bike racks and stare at the bright blue mural painted on the brick wall across from me. My vision goes out of focus and the wall blurs into the sky. *This is all a bit dramatic*, I think to myself.

Pavan comes out some time later and tells me we're going home.

'I don't want to climb when you're like this,' he says.

I make a sound, maybe a *huh*, and hope it sounds grateful. I'm silent the whole car ride home, even though I know it would be better if I said something—anything.

'I don't know what to do with this, Emma,' Pavan says when we pull up outside our house.

'I know,' I say, by which I mean *I'm sorry* and *me neither.*

'It's scary,' he tells me again.

I want to say that I'm scared, too, but I don't feel scared. I don't feel much of anything, really. The words get stuck under my tongue and I feel shame for not making this easier. It would be a whole lot less dramatic if I stopped being so quiet. *You're psycho*, I think to myself. *What are you trying to get out of this?*

That night, I stay upstairs in the bedroom and isolate from the rest of the house. Eventually, feeling comes back and I start sobbing with deep-gut shame. Pavan hears me through the floorboards and comes up to check on me.

'Sorry, sorry,' I tell him, and try to stifle my sobs.

'I'm worried about you,' he says.

I tell him not to be, that I'm fine, that I just need to be alone. Then alone becomes too much, and I phone Lifeline. I spend the first half hour of the call apologising, because they must have a real depressed person they need to speak to.

The next day, the bleeding starts. It's sunny outside, so I take my morning coffee to the courtyard and watch the magpies flit between our roof and the neighbour's fence. The air is warm against my skin, the bricks cool beneath my feet. I can see Pavan through the kitchen window, sprinkling salt onto the scrambled tofu he's making for breakfast. He's wearing a green woollen jumper, and he looks beautiful.

Our life is beautiful, I think to myself. Then I remember the Lifeline thing and stutter a laugh. How can I be catatonic one moment and at peace the next? I barely remember who I was the day before.

The more I retrace the memory of my illness, the more I come to imagine it as a kind of evil. I stretch the metaphors too far; I find new ways to pathologise myself. I have always been a little bit dramatic.

I feel stuck. I try to remember the version of myself with PMDD and come back with only fragments. I think of Robert Louis Stevenson's *The Strange Case of Dr Jekyll and Mr Hyde*: a literal interpretation of the duality of selves, the good self and the evil self. Dr Jekyll creates a serum that allows him to transform into an alter ego, Mr Hyde, through whom he can escape social expectations and indulge in the vices he so desperately longs to gratify. There is no severing of memory—

Dr Jekyll remembers perfectly the crimes of Mr Hyde—but instead a distancing of responsibility.

I cannot understand my own illness. There are days when I wake up happy and content, and I cannot fathom the anger of the night before. At other times, I wonder whether I use PMDD as an excuse: as my own serum, under the influence of which I have licence to act badly and avoid responsibility for my actions.

I am not a werewolf. There is no clean forgetting; there is no totality to my loss of control. My illness exists in a liminal place, where I am both there and not there. It is not a loss of control, rather an overwhelming compulsion; an itch I am ashamed to scratch. I don't know how to think of myself. I don't know how to think of my multitude of selves. Perhaps I am Dr Jekyll, looking for an excuse to act out. Perhaps I've always been a little bit feral, a little bit of a monster, and I'm using pathology as an excuse.

Some weeks later, driving us home from another failed climbing excursion, Pavan tries to loosen me up.

He winds his window down on Sydney Road and sticks his head out.

'I love this womaaaaan!' he shouts—as loudly as he can—into oncoming traffic, then winds the window up again.

'Go on,' he says, nudging my window down with the button. 'Yell something.'

I make a faint-hearted attempt at a *Woohoo!* and wind the window back up. I feel quiet, spent.

'That was pathetic,' he says. 'Come on, really yell it.' He wants me to dance, wants me to scream-sing along to the radio, wants me to do anything other than retreat into silence.

'I can't right now.'

He rolls the window down again, and this time he yells: 'I'm going to marry this womaaaaan!'

'Pavan,' I say. 'Not now.'

'What would Fun Emma do?'

'I don't know.'

The question renders me pathetic, sad.

'Fine, fine,' he says. I can tell he's going to keep pushing. 'Just answer me this: what would the opposite of you do right now?'

Inside me, a million bugs are rolling around, trying to crawl out any way they can. I try to imagine the opposite of me. I try to open my mind to the possibility that I'm somewhere else, someone else, someone who doesn't care about the bugs and the discomfort, someone who doesn't think that, if they were going to scream, it wouldn't be for fun, it would be for real.

'The opposite of me is skateboarding along behind the car,' I say.

'Wow, wow, wow,' he says. 'Okay. Attitude. That's something.'

'The opposite of me doesn't even use the holds at climbing, just legs it straight up the wall.'

'Damn. What's her name?'

I say the first name that comes to mind: 'Dickie.'

Pavan rolls his window down for another beat, yells: 'Dickiiiiie!' then rolls it back up.

We decide that Dickie doesn't get upset; she gets even. Dickie doesn't slide down bannisters; she slides up them. Dickie doesn't understand pain; she knows only pleasure.

I don't realise it at the time, but by creating Dickie, I've created yet another self to escape into. I've written myself into a role that allows me to act differently. I've given myself a way out, a new mask to wear. Where I've been spiralling down, Dickie spirals up. Where I've been taking this illness seriously, Dickie laughs at it.

I wasn't thinking about the life-changing possibilities of new narratives when we created Dickie, my semi-demonic skateboarding alter ego, but I do, for a while, feel a slightly different breed of frenzy.

I roll down the window, let out a scream that's more mad than playful.

16.

It's not long after Pavan moves in that the second lockdown is announced. No more climbing, no more visits from friends. On our morning walks, we feel the shift as a tangible, physical thing. The cafes are closed; there are no longer people lounging in the park.

We tell ourselves that this lockdown will be different. Better. There is a vague atmosphere of 'making the most of it' this time.

Looking for a semblance of routine, Pavan and I start virtual yoga with a couple of friends. Every day at 7.30 a.m., we open FaceTime, sync up the latest 'Yoga with Adriene' video, and follow along. On one screen: Adriene. On the other: my friends, tiny and pixellated in boxes on my phone.

By the end of each session, my chest feels deep and heavy. I dread logging on for work. I try to go for walks, for runs, but even a runner's high feels like a pyrrhic victory. I come back tired, deflated. My body is shaping itself to these lockdowns. I feel slower. My back aches. I realise how much I had relied on cycling to work, walking home from parties, dancing. All the incidental movements that made up my day have been lost. These small, intentional gestures—yoga, running—can't make up for that lack.

I start to worry about what I am eating. I've done this before, as a teenager. If premenstrual illnesses feel like gendered traps, so does this. I try to control what I eat, try to make myself smaller.

My first memory of hunger is from childhood. It is night-time, past my bedtime, and I'm telling my mum that I can't sleep because I'm hungry.

'Drink some water,' Mum tells me. She is convinced that I am not hungry—I've eaten dinner—and that I must be confusing hunger for some other feeling. She suggests thirst, then boredom, then tiredness.

'You're not hungry,' she tells me. 'You must be tired.'

I, however, am convinced that I am *starving to death*. I throw my teddy across the room and scream until I am too tired to scream anymore. Even then, the idea that feelings of hunger, thirst, boredom and tiredness could wiggle and meld imperceptibly into one another strikes something in me. Exhausted, I take the water and go to bed.

Hunger, more so than emotion, should be easy to identify. Feel hungry, eat, feel full. It enters our consciousness from an early age, starting as a bodily sensation: a wanting in the gut, a hollowness of the abdomen. Our survival depends on it. Yet, somewhere along the way, the feeling of hunger became diluted for me. Messy. Was I ravenous, or was I stressed? Did I need to eat, or was I only bored, looking for something to do? Was I elated, inspired, focused, busy—or was I hungry, and in denial?

—

In Julia Ducournau's 2016 coming-of-age-horror film, *Raw*, lifelong vegetarian Justine is forced by her older sister to eat meat as part of a cruel college hazing ritual. Justine is reluctant but dutifully swallows the rabbit kidney her sister pushes into her mouth. That night, she breaks out in a full-body rash. She vomits long, stringy hairballs. She starts to crave flesh. She loses control of her impulses, giving in to carnal desire.

When I first watched *Raw*, I couldn't look away from the image of Justine crouched in front of her fridge, eating raw chicken with her hands. At that point I had been a vegetarian for more than a decade, and vegan for a little more than five years. Justine shovelled the pink flesh into her mouth, and I was entranced. I watched her devour meat with the same breathlessness that overtook me while staring at my phone waiting for a message from a crush. It wasn't the raw meat I desired—it was the desire itself.

In my late teens, I got my first bikini wax. I felt the beautician draw long lines of wax along my labia. The hot, wet feeling dribbled down my skin and I thought, *Is this what it is to be turned on?* Then came the Velcro-like *tchhh*—and pleasure turned into warm, throbbing pain. Desire, like hunger, starts in the body. And, like hunger, I'd learned to tune it out. I begin to wonder whether it's this same obliviousness—this same willingness to tune out of my own body, my own feelings—that allowed me to ignore the cycles of my menstrual illness for so long, too.

As a teenager, I learned to mute my desire by not recognising my own queerness. I desired my friends. I wanted to—and did—kiss them. But without knowing better, I'd assumed that this desire was different from sexual desire. If it wasn't the red-hot entitlement of male desire, then what was it? Friendship? Curiosity? The desire I felt for women was different from the desire I felt for men. Not in its intensity, but in its seriousness. I *cared* what women thought of me. I cared about rejection. With men, I walked a line between not caring what they thought of me and not knowing that they thought of me at all.

Despite growing up with a feminist mother—a mother who worked, who didn't bullshit, who didn't sweat the small stuff—I'd still internalised the idea that to be a woman was to be good, to be small, to smile and be polite. I loved and loathed myself in equal parts for all the ways I was bad.

Watching *Raw*, I saw curiosity unbounded. Where I had sat with the question of desire, Justine acted. She followed her impulses: however unwilling, however feral, however monstrous. I place Justine within a lineage of classical female monsters, next to Medusa, Charybdis and Scylla. I think of Justine as another way to view these monsters, another way to tell the story of this curse.

In some ways, it is obvious why eating is a frequent subject in the horror genre: we do not want to be eaten. Still, time and time again, it is specifically *women* who devour and become monstrous. I can think of few narratives featuring women quenching their appetites that are not coded as horror. No wonder it's when I feel like my most monstrous self that I begin to fear food. How can any woman not fear her own hunger when the act of satiation is deemed so terrific?

Where Justine's male classmates enact desire by forcing freshmen to dress like 'sluts' and engaging in sweaty bacchanalian raves, Justine's hunger is outsized. When pushed into a bathroom to make out with one of her male classmates, she bites off his lip: an act of monstrous desire. She goes home, ravenously horny, and fucks her roommate. The scene is uncomfortable to watch. It is about her desire, not his.

'Horror films offer a fantasy space for women whose bodies betray them,' writes Australian essayist Rebecca Harkins-Cross in her piece 'Only Women Bleed'. 'When the female flesh invariably exceeds its bounds, it may become a site of transcendence, even resistance.'

Again: monsters as spirals, inwards or out. In horror, the pull goes both ways—outwards, into a desirous force that could swallow the world, or inwards, into the panic of being consumed by one's own appetites. I write about *Raw* because there is something in Justine's monstrosity that I feel within myself—want within myself. I want her desire. I want to want. To be a woman is to be a monster. To want at all is to want too much.

One of the only studies into long-term starvation is the Minnesota Starvation Experiment, run just after World War II. In that study, a group of young white men underwent voluntary starvation to help scientists better understand how to help a person recover from long periods of extreme hunger. There have been no other studies quite like it; no ethics board would approve such a thing today.

The subjects were chosen carefully: they were all physically and mentally healthy, and sociable enough to get along with others. Of the two hundred men who volunteered, only 36 made the cut.

For six months, the men were put on a semi-starvation diet. They grew gaunt. Their strength diminished. Their body temperatures cooled, their heart rates lowered. Many lost their sex drive. The men started fantasising about food. It was all they could talk about. They would read about food, then savour every bite of their two meals a day. They coddled their food as though it were a baby, licked their plates clean. It entered their dreams. They were obsessed.

When the time came to start eating again, the men had lost control of their appetites. They ate and ate, unable to feel full. One man ate so much he needed his stomach pumped. After such a long period of denial, the men did not remember what it was like to feel satiated. It took months before their eating habits returned to normal. Eventually, though, normalcy did return.

Of course, from the Minnesota Starvation Experiment we better understand the effects of starvation on men. And like much medical research, the findings of the experiment have been transposed onto the female body, as though, once more, to be a woman is simply to be a smaller man.

What happens when a woman is starved? Once more, without scientific literature to turn to, I turn to literature instead.

In a polar narrative to Ducournau's *Raw*, the protagonist of Han Kang's *The Vegetarian*, Yeong-hye, begins her journey towards a denial of sustenance by refusing to eat meat after a series of distressing dreams. Her quiet act is obscene in the eyes of her husband and family. Soon, Yeong-hye gives up food altogether, attempting to erase the violent parts of her body ('hand, foot, tongue, gaze') and become plant instead. Her body horror comes not from the destruction of other bodies, but the diminishment of her own. She is surrendered to an inpatient hospital. No one—not her husband, her father, her sister—can understand why she refuses to eat.

Both *The Vegetarian* and *Raw* use meat to position women's desire as chronic. Kang's heroine becomes pathological in her desire to inflict no harm; Ducournau's becomes pathological in her inability to avoid it.

Each time I have been to a new doctor and told them that I am vegan, they have requested a blood test. This is standard protocol, I am sure. Besides, I am lucky: every blood test has come back fine. I have never been anaemic. But I have grown intimate with the idea that it's this choice—my veganism, my desire not to harm animals—that might be one variable as to why I am unwell or unhappy.

Through each blood test—through telling each doctor that it's probably not my iron, and them testing just to be sure—I have become familiar with the notion that it is possibly worse and harder for those who menstruate to go without meat than it is for those who don't. Yet, through a decade of veganism, I have also become familiar with the ways that avoiding meat is viewed as feminine. Manly men, for whatever reason, need meat.

Raw is a film about female desire, but it is also a film about meat. In an early scene, Justine—then vegetarian—makes the radical claim that an animal's internal landscape could be just as complicated as a woman's.

'So you're saying that a raped monkey feels as much as a raped woman?' another student asks with disgust.

'Yes,' says Justine, drawing on a trope that has existed since Cartesian times: what difference is there between a woman and an animal? Unlike Descartes, Justine doesn't use this comparison to reduce the female experience, but to acknowledge the wealth of desire and pain and experience that exists beyond what is human. What is desire—what is hunger—if not an animal impulse? Meat and vegetarianism become symbols of desire and the suppression of desire respectively. This desire is not meant to be feminine. I see meat tied to stories of men as hunters: meat is supposed to make us bigger, stronger. In a culture that doesn't particularly value women who are big—or strong, or hunters—it is easy, I think, for stories of women devouring meat to become stories of women who want too much.

I list burger joints in my head: Brother Burger, Mr Burger, Royale Brothers, Rockwell and Sons, Danny's, Andrew's, Bad Boys, Fat Bob's, Fat Jak's, Hungry Jack's. Betty's Burgers is the exception: a fifties pin-up style burger bar that serves low-carb patties between lettuce-leaf buns.

During the lockdowns, I gain weight. Most of the time, this is fine. Then, in the days before my period, when I am most animal, most out of control, I feel as though my body is dissolving into mush. I fear my own desire. I fear my want of food, my want of comfort, my want of support. I fear that I am like Justine: ravenous, unbridled, monstrous for transcending the meekness of my femininity. I think all this through the language of my animal brain: *too much, too demanding, too greedy, a slut.*

I don't want to be this kind of monster, so I begin to avoid food.

I think of emotions as animal sensations: pleasure, pain, arousal, calm. From our animal selves, we write and rewrite the story behind our feeling, express it in our own emotional vocabulary: anger, hurt, desire, love, joy.

When it comes to diagnosing this internal feeling—to putting sensation into words—I am inaccurate and messy. I write my body a fiction.

Hunger, like emotion, is a transient feeling. The physical sensation of hunger—discomfort, pain—only lasts in the body for around twenty minutes. Usually, we acknowledge the hunger and feed it. However, when we ignore our hunger, the feeling *will* go away. But the need for food will not. Our hunger will return, and return.

When I read about the biological fact of hunger's transience, it's usually framed as a positive thing: *Don't worry! It will pass*, the internet reassures me. There is a difference between *true hunger*, the need to eat, and *appetite*, the desire to eat, whether out of boredom, tiredness, stress, or simply being a four-year-old girl who does not want to go to bed.

Online, article after article echoes my mother: *Thirst can often be confused with hunger, so keep yourself hydrated by drinking plenty of water.*

I think of *The Vegetarian*, how Yeong-hye believed that she could live off water alone, how she pushed her needs back, back, until she felt that she could dig her body into the soil.

It is possible to acknowledge the physical sensation of hunger without satiating it. I doubt I am equipped to handle my needs and desires this way. I keep putting up barriers against them, fearing the flood that will come when they fall. I wonder if I would fear my own hunger less if, instead of assuring myself that it will pass, I chose to eat, and convinced myself that eating would leave me satisfied.

Despite resenting narratives of mood swings, irrational women and crazed biologies—gendered narratives, intended to diminish—I adhere to them. Only as an adult have I realised that my inability to feel—or rather, diagnose—hunger is connected to other denials of my body.

If I was unprepared to identify my own desire, my own appetite, my own hunger, how could I anticipate the causal relationship between my monstrous feelings and the flux of hormones I experience each month?

I stumble across whole subgenres of film connecting a woman's sexuality with cannibalistic desires and flesh-craving tendencies. In *Teeth*, a young woman learns that she has *vagina dentata*—a condition that results in her vagina biting the dick off any man who tries to force himself onto her. In Diablo Cody's *Jennifer's Body*, Adam Brody attempts to sacrifice a virgin to make his band famous. But his virgin, Jennifer, has lied about her sexual history, and the ritual turns her into a boy-eating demon instead. Both films express desire against a patriarchal backdrop. Men's actions make monsters out of these women. In this setting, desire becomes revenge.

Jennifer's Body, now a cult classic, was a commercial flop. Megan Fox, who plays the titular Jennifer, had just wrapped up *Transformers*, where she plays a hot, sexy romantic interest. The marketing of *Jennifer's Body* leaned into that angle: *how* hot *is Megan Fox?* The film is about demonic revenge on men who only want a woman for her body, but the marketing focused on one thing: Megan's body. The boys who turned up at the cinema saw a monstrous woman with monstrous desires. They hated it. It was uncomfortable to watch. It was about her desire, not theirs.

Jennifer's Body and *Raw* feature similar horrific tropes: a bloody transformation, devouring raw chicken from the fridge, vomiting sludge, preening in the mirror, an insatiable desire for flesh. They are also intertwined for another reason: both are coming-of-age narratives.

In a 2021 review for her 'Uterine Horror' column in the indie horror publication *Certified Forgotten*, author and film critic Molly Henery connects Jennifer's monstrosity with her menstrual cycle. 'For a majority of the time,' she writes, 'Jennifer is her usual succubus self. Then comes the time of renewal. Just like people who menstruate shed their uterine lining in a painful, bloody process to renew the uterus, Jennifer must rejuvenate herself in a similarly violent fashion. The only difference: it's the blood and guts of teenage boys that is shed in Jennifer's cycle.'

For most of the month, Pavan and I are in love. We're best friends. We laugh and fuck and dance around our room together. The rest of the time, I fear that I am devouring him: that I am the monster and he will be my sacrifice.

—

After three months of observing my cycle, I can see my duality of selves clearly. I am fine 70 per cent of the time. The data is there, in front of me, written by me, and yet it continues to surprise me. I am happy, occasionally stressed, occasionally tired. I had assumed that I was forgetting how bad things were, not how good.

Even with these happy days, PMDD seems to always be looming around the corner, or to have only recently passed. In my app, the five or six days before my period are marked with cartoonish storm clouds. My mood drops. The pits of my knees ache. My breasts are tender. I am irritable, aching, depressed and combative.

Outside of the luteal phase, there is only one major change in my moods: the day one of our family dogs dies.

I keep turning to film and fiction as though it will understand this illness for me. I long for something better. I want to write my own way out of this illness. Perhaps I am regurgitating these stories of monsters because I feel that by writing through the mythologies and taboos that surround periods, I will somehow write around them. My goal is to write something more truthful about menstruation.

My fear is that, by writing honestly about the pain of premenstruation, I will reinforce the taboos and mythologies that reduce options for women within the medical system. Already, so many of the medications we use do not take female biology into account.

Menstruating women are excluded from medical trials for the very reason of having periods. The variables in their hormonal cycle are deemed *difficult to study*. The period is irrational—unscientific. Safer, I suppose, to test on men. But if periods are an irrational variable, they are my irrational variable; they are a quarter of the world's irrational variable. People with periods are twice as likely to experience adverse effects to medication: nausea, headaches, depression, cognitive deficits, seizures, hallucinations, agitation and cardiac anomalies.

In tracking my cycle and formalising my own diagnosis, I feel this more than ever. I am wrong for the very reasons they refuse to study me. I am malfunctioning in all the expected ways.

I make a virtual appointment with my GP and show her my baseline data. She's unsurprised.

'Usually, we would treat PMDD with antidepressants,' she tells me, echoing my last visit.

I don't tell her that I have started worrying about food again. That I am looking for some semblance of control. I'm not sure why antidepressants frighten me so much, only that I fear the weight gain, the sexual dysfunction, the withdrawal afterwards, the idea of taking a medication all the time for an illness that only affects me for a few days each month.

'I've read about a new version of the pill,' I say instead. The pill seems less intense, better suited to everyday use. 'It's supposed to help with PMDD.'

She agrees to put me on it, but seems annoyed that I won't agree to the antidepressants.

So, I tell her that I am concerned about side effects: sexual dysfunction, weight gain. Sexual dysfunction sounds like the worst version of not coming I can think of.

'Weight gain is usually minimal,' she says. 'And besides, you're probably too depressed to have much of a sex drive anyway.'

I want to tell her that two things can be true: I can be sick, and I can want to fuck.

17.

In the opening of *The Birth of the Clinic* (1963), Michel Foucault describes two separate instances of medical observation. In the first example, an eighteenth-century doctor treats a hysterical patient by prescribing her 'baths, ten or twelve hours a day, for ten whole months'. The doctor, Pierre Pomme, observes as the patient begins to dissolve, whole parts of her sloughing off like soft, dead skin. Pomme describes this process: 'membranous tissues like pieces of damp parchment . . . peel away with some slight discomfort, and these were passed daily with the urine; the right ureter also peeled away and came out whole in the same way'. His descriptions read like fantasy, or poetry. I can hardly hold on to each image. I can't view her disintegration as real.

Foucault compares Pomme's observations with those of another doctor, Bayle, working less than a century later, who describes with clinical precision the dissection of the membranes of the brain:

> Their outer surface, which is next to the arachnoidian layer of the dura mater, adheres to this layer, sometimes very lightly, when they can be separated easily, sometimes very firmly and

> tightly, in which case it can be very difficult to detach them. Their internal surface is only contiguous with the arachnoid, and is in no way joined to it . . . The false membranes are often transparent, especially when they are very thin; but usually they are white, grey, or red in colour . . .

I've excerpted only some of the text Foucault uses to illustrate the point he makes: the ways that we talk about medicine are not static. Where Pomme describes a woman dissolving in the manner of a fairytale, Bayle draws our eyes towards the visible, nameable and quantifiable aspects of the human body. Both doctors are writing from direct observation, and yet shifts in medical and scientific culture have created a gulf between the two examples. As Foucault writes, 'For us, [the difference between observations] is total, because each of Bayle's words, with its qualitative precision, directs our gaze into a world of constant visibility, while Pomme, lacking any perceptual base, speaks to us in the language of fantasy.'

Naming an illness can affect the reality of an illness, the experience of it. Foucault argues for some scepticism towards the purported objectivity of modern medicine. From within a scientific era, it's near impossible to see its flaws: how can we be sure that, with fewer than one hundred years of advancement separating them, one doctor's gaze is so unquestionably accurate, and another's so fantastically wrong? How can we be sure that there is not some truth within the now implausible fact of disintegration that Pomme describes? Both doctors wrote what they observed. It's the nature of looking, of naming, of observing, that seems to have changed.

—

The further back I move through time, looking for women who share this illness, the more disparate our language for it becomes. One hundred years ago, PMDD would have sat somewhere within the muck of *hysteria*. While Sandie and Christine *may* have had PMDD, their doctors called it premenstrual syndrome, or tension. PMS or PMT, a series of confusing acronyms that jumble around to mean something like *moodiness before your period*.

Today, the differences between PMS and PMDD are both subtle and absolute. While PMS is a catch-all for the symptoms that might precede a period—bloating, tenderness, irritability—PMDD has strict diagnostic criteria, as outlined in the most recent *Diagnostic and Statistical Manual of Mental Disorders*.

The DSM-V lists a range of symptoms that a person must exhibit in specific combinations in order to be diagnosed with PMDD. These symptoms must be present during the luteal phase of the menstrual cycle and resolve within a few days of menstruation. The criteria listed by the DSM-V are broad, and include symptoms such as 'mood swings', 'a sense of being overwhelmed or out of control', 'marked irritability or anger', 'lethargy', 'insomnia' and 'physical symptoms such as breast tenderness or swelling; joint or muscle pain, a sensation of "bloating" or weight gain'.

While many of these symptoms overlap with PMS, it's the severity of them that distinguishes PMDD. For a person to be diagnosed with PMDD, symptoms must cause 'clinically significant distress', interfering with someone's ability to go about daily life, maintain relationships, go to school or function at work.

Only two menstrual cycles need to be accurately observed to meet the diagnostic criteria. I have three. Each month, my moods swing, I lash out, I can't work, I sleep during the day. I map my symptoms against the diagnostic criteria and meet them all. While I've long known I have PMDD, this is the first time it seems obvious and clear-cut. By tracking a baseline—by diagnosing myself in a less haphazard way than I had been diagnosed in 2015—I've perhaps confirmed the obvious. But I've also moved myself away from the language of fantasy—of assumptions and guesses—and towards something more scientific and rational.

For me, the difference I experienced on completing this diagnostic process was total. It reduced the space for fantasy and doubt. Before I could clearly name the illness, I externalised it. I felt distressed, uneasy, uncontrolled and directionless. The world was wrong; I was wrong; it didn't matter. It all swirled around me like unknowable, floating matter. Once I could view my diagnosis within the clinical lens of modern medicine, my gaze turned entirely inwards. I was ill, and this was how. I stared directly into the abyss and now, with naming as knowing, the abyss stared back. This illness was chronic. Instead of imagining it as a monster, or fantasy, I imagined it as the rational hands of a clock, looping round and back around. I could expect to feel this way one out of every four weeks for the next 25 years of my life, give or take. Though the experience of my illness had changed little, the weight of it had multiplied.

I could not live like this, I decided.

18.

I'm reading about resilience. I want to learn how to build it and to understand why I don't have it. The days when I can do the work, when I am motivated and driven, start to feel few and far between. I want to be useful. I want to stop endlessly chasing my own tail. Increasingly, work feels looming and meaningless. I sit and stare at the screen, doing only the tasks I know I can report back on in my end-of-day update. Those are the days I look most productive. I feel that something is wrong inside of me. I have malfunctioned. I feel that I am useless, that I will never work again.

Before modern capitalism, the word *productive* referred to plants and fields, not people. In *The Protestant Ethic and the Spirit of Capitalism*, German sociologist Max Weber outlines how, prior to the seventeenth century, most people worked with the ultimate goals being subsistence and leisure, not the accumulation of wealth. It wasn't until the Protestant church was able to convince people of the moral imperative of hard work that our conception of productivity changed. Work became a calling. Discipline was virtuous. Earning more money than necessary, and spending it wisely, showed dedication, faith and moral value.

I've tried to reject capital as a measure of my own success. *I work to live*, I tell myself. *I don't live to work*. When I was offered a promotion at my last workplace, I turned down the pay increase and negotiated a shorter working week instead. Same money, fewer hours. Slowly, I've been building myself a warm nest egg of time. Time to write, time to make things, time with the people I love.

Now, time feels meaningless. I am meaningless.

I want to feel virtuous, dedicated. I think that if I am going to be miserable, I should at least be making money. I should be getting something useful out of this lockdown.

The pill I ask to go on is called Yaz. It's a combination pill, which means that it contains both drospirenone and ethinyl estradiol—synthetic forms of progesterone and oestrogen. By taking a constant stream of hormones, I hope that the ebbs and flows of my cycle will end. Online, on a PMDD forum, someone describes Yaz as a lifesaver. I look at the pill and think that it could be a way out, a way to stop tracing the erratic spirals my body makes.

I'm hoping that my mood will stabilise, and I won't be such a mess anymore.

In the first half of the twentieth century, Margaret Sanger, the founder of Planned Parenthood, was searching for a 'magic pill'—a pill that would prevent pregnancy and could be taken without a man's knowledge. She wanted to end cycles of oppression for women, to liberate women from the fate of forced motherhood, to end the downward spiral that begins, for many women, with tissue growing in the womb. Most urgently, she wanted to give women, especially poor and working-class women, a choice when it came to childbirth. She was disillusioned with the slow progress of democracy and legalisation, asking herself whether 'any male politician could understand of the wrongs inflicted upon poor working women'. Her solution was birth control.

Sanger couldn't invent the pill alone. She needed a team: someone with money to fund the project, a biologist to do the research, and a doctor with enough charisma to get the whole thing through a conservative government.

Over the course of the 1950s, Sanger pulled together that very team. She recruited Katharine D. McCormick, a lifelong feminist who had inherited $35 million after the death of her husband, to fund the project. The two then approached biologist Gregory Goodwin Pincus. At the time, Pincus was on the fringe of the scientific community. In 1934, he had successfully completed the first ever in-vitro fertilisation of rabbits—a feat that horrified much of the scientific establishment. *The New York Times* called him 'Dr. Frankenstein'. Harvard revoked his tenure. The public, made uneasy by the seemingly sterile nature of test-tube babies, derided him. For Sanger and McCormick, he was their best hope.

Pincus's goal was singular: to break every component of human and animal nature down to its biological make-up. He was uninterested in the social ramifications of his research. He did not care for feminism, nor social liberation. 'I am against women having sexual freedom,' he once said. 'But I hasten to add that I am also opposed to sexual freedom among men.'

With money and brains behind her, Sanger was almost there. But to get her project over the final hurdles—drug trials, legalisation, social approval—she needed someone who could sell it. Sanger brought on 'the good doctor', John Rock, a Harvard-educated physician who was attractive, well-spoken and—critically—Catholic. Sanger approached him for help conducting (and getting approval for) contraceptive medical trials. Rock had a wealth of experience conducting medical trials at the Harvard Medical School–affiliated Free Hospital for Women, including testing synthetic hormones on many of his low-income patients. Unlike Pincus, Rock was interested in science for its social possibilities. By the time Sanger approached him, Rock had set his sights on the issue of overpopulation. He was interested in finding a way to curb population growth without betraying Catholic doctrine, which prohibited artificial contraception. Rock cared less about giving women agency, and more about preventing women who he viewed as unfit—black women, brown women, uneducated women, disabled women—from having children.

'People like to have babies,' Rock would say later in life. 'And this is particularly so among primitive peoples.'

The feminist, the wealthy widow, the mad scientist, the Catholic hunk. Together, they formed a Cluedo board of characters, each playing their part to ensure the contraceptive pill came to fruition.

—

The first two days are the worst.

The morning after I start taking the pill, I don't move—I just lie on the floor. I post a greeting in the work chat. We don't have our usual morning meeting: my boss is away. I try to muster the ability to move, to do anything, but I'm glued to the floor. I think that I have lost any resilience I might once have had. I don't know how to respect myself when I'm like this, prostrate and static on the floor.

Pavan comes in to check on me and sees that I haven't moved. 'Aren't you supposed to be working?' he asks.

'I am,' I say.

My laptop is open on the ground next to me. Every now and again I flick the trackpad to keep my status *online.* At midday, I send the team a message that I'm going to lunch. I continue to lie on the floor.

'Do you want to go for a walk?' Pavan asks. I don't.

I remain on the floor, curling my body into something foetal, and wait for time to pass.

Pincus was interested in how the human experience—our feelings and decisions—could be explained by chemical interactions and hormonal impulses. When he began working on the pill, he started with a biological truth: a mammal could not become pregnant once it was already pregnant. He started looking at ways of tricking the body into believing that it was pregnant. He started testing on mice and rabbits, injecting them with pregnancy hormones. Their bodies were pumped with oestrogen and progesterone, then they were left to mate and eat and live. Later, Pincus dissected their ovaries and scraped their fallopian tubes for evidence of life or eggs. Once he had perfected birth control for rabbits, Pincus began to test on humans, too.

That's where the Catholic hunk came in. Beginning in 1954, John Rock ran a series of medical trials at the Free Hospital, where for years he had treated a largely poor and working-class population. There he taught women about the 'rhythm' method of contraception: the only method of contraception that was legal and Pope-approved at the time. The rhythm method relied on only having sex during times when the body naturally produced high levels of progesterone. When he started trials of Pincus's progesterone pill, he believed it to be an extension of this method. Rock saw little moral difference in prolonging that safe period with artificial progesterone.

Rock and Pincus wanted the pill to mirror a 'natural cycle'. The more similarities they could draw between the pill as a method of contraception and the rhythm method, the better. They wanted to keep the appearance of a period, so that conservatives (and the Pope) could look at the pill and see it as something natural, moral and safe. This moral concern was the sole rationale behind the pill's three-weeks-on, one-week-off schedule.

Even with these appeals to nature, too many women dropped out of John Rock's early Free Hospital trials. Of the 60 women enrolled in the program, 30 withdrew, citing disturbing side effects, or an overly demanding routine. Of the women remaining, 15 per cent still showed signs of ovulation. These women were not rabbits, and Pincus was unsatisfied with the results. The project's benefactor, the wealthy widow McCormick, was also displeased that so many women had dropped out. Frustrated, she wrote in a letter that she longed for a *'cage' of ovulating females to experiment with.*

By the end of lunch on Tuesday I want to die. There is no spectacular drama to this. There is no specific rationale. I simply start planning how I might end my life. I write a list in my journal of how I will divide the few assets to my name. I debate quitting my job. My thought process is something like this: if I am going to kill myself, I don't need to work. If I am not going to kill myself, I need the money. I am not completely gone. Somewhere inside me is survival instinct enough to know there should be choice beyond these binaries, but I am not well enough to search for them.

I message my boss's boss to say that I am unwell.

Is it urgent? she asks.

I don't know what to make of the question.

Yes, I type back after a while. *I think it is.*

She tells me to make a list of the projects I am working on, along with their status, to hand over to my boss when she returns. I write the list from my bedroom floor. My breath is short and sharp. I can't breathe so much as gasp. As soon as I send her my notes, I log off and lie back down on the floor.

I take one week off work, then another. For some reason, I keep taking the pill.

—

Eventually, John Rock helped McCormick find her cage of ovulating women. He expanded his trials, looking for women who were already being considered for forced sterilisation projects by the United States government. Two locations proved promising. The first was an asylum in Massachusetts, where he could test the drug on 'chronic psychotic patients'. The second was in Puerto Rico, where their team would be free to test on black and brown women with little government intervention.

There were few barriers to approval within the mental asylum's walls. The director of the hospital was another Harvard alum, who was pleased to have more physicians on hand in a too-big, overcrowded hospital. No forms needed to be signed. In exchange for the asylum's cooperation, McCormick offered to pay for some of the wards' rooms to be painted.

Not long after starting the first set of trials in Massachusetts, in the summer of 1955, Gregory Pincus headed for Puerto Rico. On paper, the island seemed like the perfect place to continue the trials: densely populated, it had no anti-birth-control laws, and the team could rely on government support. When Pincus arrived, he was impressed by the wide range of birth-control clinics across the island. Here, it would be possible to access all the women they needed, without political interference. Within this 'cage' of ovulating females, Pincus had another point to prove: if poor, uneducated Puerto Rican women could take the pill, then it would be simple enough for the rest of America to take, too.

Though the medical team tried to keep the instructions clear, they were ineffective, perhaps poorly communicated, and mistakes were inevitable. Each participant was given a bottle of twenty pills and told to take one per day until the bottle was finished. One woman went home and took all the pills at once. Another gave them out to her friends.

In the first Puerto Rican trial, 80 per cent of participants quit. Some cited disapproving husbands, some just stopped showing up, and at least 25 women withdrew due to harsh side effects. Pincus was unconcerned: he had plenty more women to choose from. By 1956, 221 women had participated in the trial. Seventeen women became pregnant. *They're just not following instructions*, he told McCormick in a letter.

Pincus began to search for more patients. He hired a woman to walk through a neighbourhood that was so poor and crowded that there were no sewers and no toilets, and barely enough room between houses to move, and take a census of the women there. *How many children do you have? Are you sterilised?*

There was no shortage of new participants to be found. When one woman quit due to headaches, nausea, breakthrough bleeding, a new woman signed up. Many of these women were so poor and so desperate to avoid pregnancy that they continued to take the pill despite its side effects. Yet the drop-out rate remained high throughout the trials. Eventually, Pincus stopped talking about the women at all—instead of *130 participants*, he wrote of *1279 menstrual cycles*. He severed his research from the experiences of these women, separated their cycles from their lives, in an effort to make his research more rational, scientific, controlled.

—

I make a remote appointment with my GP to ask for a medical certificate for the time I have taken off work. She asks me if I have a plan, meaning, do I know how I am going to kill myself. I tell her that I don't know how I'll do it, then start thinking of ways I might. She writes me a note for the second week off work, the time my sick leave won't cover but my annual leave will.

I'm unmotivated to act. I want to lie in bed and waste away. I stare at the ceiling all morning, unable to do anything, wondering if I'm putting it on. If I just changed my mindset, perhaps all these dramatics would fade away. I think about dying again, then tell myself I'm doing it for attention. I want to use all the work leave I have left. I can't imagine these feelings going away.

Pavan tries to get me to watch TV with him, but instead of relaxing me it makes me panic. I feel that I am melting into nothing. The lockdown seems endless. I don't know what to do with this time. I still lack the resilience to get through it. At night, I take a Valium and feel better for a moment.

I sleep for most of the day and am still able to sleep through the night. I feel slow, on mute. I keep thinking that Pavan deserves better than this. This depression isn't solitary: everyone is depressed. One friend has to hide the kitchen knives from her housemate, because she won't stop self-harming. Another friend goes totally silent, stops responding to messages, drops out of all virtual activities. When someone walks past his house to check on him, he opens the door for a minute, says, 'It's cold,' then shuts the door again.

Pavan is the only person I know who seems to be okay. Every lockdown inspires a new screenplay idea, a new story, a new sketch, a new song, a new business idea. They don't get finished, but perhaps the start of something is enough to survive on.

Five women died in the Puerto Rican pill trials. More than 65 per cent of the women complained of at least one side effect. Some 17 per cent came forward with complaints of severe nausea, bloating and vomiting. Pincus dismissed these complaints, called them psychosomatic. Instead of listening to these women, he wrote their symptoms off as the 'emotional super-activity of Puerto Rican women'.

The pill's invention was revelatory for women. Yet the process behind its invention is revealing, too. There are ways in which women are expected to suffer, in which their discomfort is normalised. When given a choice between discomfort and pregnancy, the choice seems simple. I fear that women are used to choosing between two poorly dealt hands.

Ultimately, the pill's early side effects were deemed minuscule in comparison to its benefits. Later, when male contraceptives first reached the clinical-trials stage, these same side effects caused an independent safety-review board to cut the trials short.

I have taken the pill before. When I was fifteen, a dermatologist wanted to treat my acne with a drug called Roaccutane, which is notorious for causing birth defects. At the time, I was years away from having sex at all, let alone the kind that could get me pregnant. When I tried to tell her that I wasn't having sex, she didn't believe me. I was one of any number of young women who might lie to her mum and her doctor.

'You would have to get an abortion if you became pregnant,' she told me. 'What are you using for contraception?'

Unsure how to answer, I shrugged. 'My face, I guess?'

'We'll need to put you on the pill,' she said, unamused.

She called it *the pill* when she meant *the oral contraceptive*, because we all knew what she meant, anyway. What I didn't know was that *the pill* was a combination of oestrogen and progesterone. What I didn't know was the effect these hormones would have on my body, on my brain.

I didn't know the history of the pill. I didn't know that its founding was fuelled not only by a dream of women's liberation, but by racism, eugenics and religious doctrine, too. I didn't know that doctors had assured women the drug was safe, and yet some of them had died. I didn't know any of this, and I didn't even think to ask, because it was just the pill, and the pill was normal.

When I left the dermatologist's office, she made me sign a long list of waivers about the risks of Roaccutane. Birth defects, bloody urine, burning eyes, peeling skin, thinning hair, changes in behaviour, suicidal ideation. I didn't sign anything for the pill.

Within a few months, my skin had cleared and I'd started throwing up after most meals. When my mum found out, she made an appointment with a children's psychologist in Clifton Hill, across the road from the dermatologist. I never once thought to blame the pill.

I know that the pill will stop me from ovulating. I know that it will stop me from getting pregnant. I now know that the pill I am taking contains a mix of oestrogen and progesterone, and that this is—somehow—supposed to be better.

When I take the pill, the loops and spirals of ovulation are supposed to stop.

19.

Two weeks into starting the pill, I check in with my doctor again. I feel further from the edge than I was at first, but still shaken and low. Again she suggests antidepressants. I feel anxiety swell in me anew. What if another medication puts me back on that same rollercoaster? What if I end up depressed and sluggish and delirious all the time, instead of just for a certain period each month? When I tell her that I am nervous about taking more medications, she writes a referral to a psychiatrist. After the first line, she starts calling me Emily. She writes, *I'm concerned that Emily's reluctance is probably harming her.*

I stumble across a photo of Gregory Pincus at Harvard University in 1932. In it, he's wearing a dirty lab coat, and there are dark rings around his eyes. He holds a rabbit in his arms like it's a baby, one hand supporting the back, the other supporting the head. He's looking down at the rabbit tenderly. I think the rabbit is dead.

Pavan holds me at night. I am miserable and despondent. He tells me that it will be okay, kisses me on the lips. The moment feels warm, tender. All I can think is that it's a nice moment for us to share before I die.

I go back to the asset-division list in my journal and note the potential beneficiaries of my superannuation. I think of my friends who will be sad, and how the little money I have might help to make their sadness go away. I think of who will take my plants, my books, and write it all down.

I plan how I will do it, and how I might be found.

The next day, I message my mum and ask if I can borrow Harry, the surviving family dog, for a few days. We're not allowed to meet, but she agrees anyway. We cross over in a park between our houses and walk together for a few minutes.

'Shouldn't we be worried?' I ask. She reminds me that my licence still has her address on it, that legally I'm still part of her household. I want to cry. This is the same woman who once refused to round up by a single minute in my logbook when I was learning to drive, saying it was breaking the rules.

When we get home, Harry seems confused by the new arrangement and spends the morning looking around the share house for my dad. When he realises that I'm the only person he knows here, he follows me everywhere.

'We should keep him forever,' Pavan says. 'You're so much happier.'

I enjoy our daily walks more than Harry does. Within fifteen minutes, Harry tries to steer me back home, back inside where it's warm and we can nap. He's a strange dog, with human eyes and a stiff-legged walk. When I take him off his lead, he walks along beside me. I try to avoid other dogs, knowing he'll snap if they show too much interest.

'This side, Harry,' I tell him when we walk past another dog, and even though we haven't trained him to do so, he listens.

At night, he sleeps at the end of our bed—an arrangement my parents would be disgusted by.

After a week, Mum messages me to ask for the dog back.

'Your dad won't admit it,' she says, 'but he misses him too much.'

We meet at a park again. When Harry sees my dad, he runs towards him without so much as a glance in my direction.

Back at home, I show Pavan which compartment the laundry liquid goes in. When I try to write in the study, he interrupts to ask me where something is. I wish that I could forget the layout of my own house. I wish I could empty myself of everything I know. I wish I could forget about work, about the chores that need to be done, forget about the details.

Instead, I show Pavan where the keys are (desk), where the KeepCups are (pantry), where the juice is (fridge).

I don't know how to stop sweating the small stuff.

—

Case numbers continue to rise, and we all know the lockdown will be extended. When there are more than seven hundred unexplained cases in the state, we enter a new stage of lockdown—Stage 4. Another six weeks. By comparison, the early lockdowns look like jokes. Now, we cannot go more than five kilometres from our homes. A curfew is put in place between 8 p.m. and 5 a.m. We're allowed an hour of exercise outdoors, once per day, either alone or with one other member of our household. No more walks with friends. One person from a household can visit the grocery store. Other than these reasons, I have no excuse to leave the house.

The night the new rules are announced I feel so panicked that I take a Valium to calm down.

I hear about friends-of-friends taking their own lives. The day before the new rules take effect, Pavan and I see groups gathered in the park on our afternoon walk. More people than usual. As we pass, we realise that they are listening in to a funeral. They are all young, in their twenties, perhaps two dozen people all up, all distantly huddled in twos and threes. There are restrictions on funeral attendance, too.

A friend of mine, driven stir-crazy by the solitude, bends the rules and spends whole days walking along Merri Creek alone. They FaceTime friends, call their parents. They're not afraid of getting caught breaking the one-hour time limit: who would be watching for long enough to know?

Two of our single friends pretend to date each other, call each other *intimate partners*, just so they can see another person.

I read about a police bust on a house party. The police were alerted by an abnormally large KFC order, and followed the delivery driver to the drop-off address. People hid in closets, trying not to get caught, the story goes.

Pavan and I continue our morning walks. The park is empty. Around the playground and the skate park, most of the benches are taped off. We see police officers on horses. They don't stop us, though I see them question another couple, asking if they live together. The couple pull out their house keys to show that they match.

On the pill, my mood is now steady, though I am no longer happy. I am constantly low.

After another two weeks, I feel stable enough to know that I am not going to kill myself. Not actually, not for real.

My GP tells me that it was probably just the initial spike in progesterone that got me. It should have levelled out now, she says. I take the pill religiously every morning. I am scared to miss a day, scared that a single missed dose will cause a slip-and-spike that could send me straight back to day one, comatose with depression.

I ask work for more time off, and they tell me I'm out of leave. Personal and annual. My role is being subsidised by the government's JobKeeper scheme to prevent COVID-related layoffs, so I ask about taking additional leave and using the money they receive from that to cover my rent, but they don't have clear answers. They say something about how they would have to keep it to cover the costs of rehiring someone. I don't think this is true. I've updated fact sheet after fact sheet on topics like this. But those fact sheets don't take into account how useless I have been, and I no longer trust myself to know the truth.

I am hollow and fragile. I am too tired to argue. I hate myself for being so lazy. I want to sleep in, stare at the ceiling, go for afternoon walks, not worry about my rent being paid. I feel ashamed of these feelings; I don't want to be a dole bludger, a mooch. I'm harder on myself than I would be on anyone else.

20.

When I return to work, my boss arranges a one-on-one meeting to catch me up. She tells me that she is disappointed by the way I left things before the break, then asks me what she can do to make work more manageable. I'm not sure what to say. I don't know how to help her help me. There's a world in which I tell her that I'm unfit for work during *that time of the month.* I'm irrational and unreliable. I could set up a new schedule to work more when I'm ovulating, less when I'm luteal. I know I would be more productive, work harder. But I still feel the threads of what I have to live for as tender, fragile things. I can't imagine spending the only happy days I have at work, and my only free time in the pits. Besides, the pill has put an end to that cycle. I don't even have the predictability of my own biology anymore. I'm just a little bruised all over, all the time.

When I can't offer a solution to make work easier, my boss suggests more check-ins. We already check in three times a day: a half-hour 'stand-up' meeting in the morning, plus a pre-lunch check-in and an end-of-day progress report. We already have fortnightly team meetings on top of the stand-ups, plus fortnightly one-on-ones. There's no lack of check-ins, but I'm in no state to say this. I feel guilty, criminal, like I deserve to be watched, monitored, judged. I agree to turn my fortnightly check-in into a weekly one.

She asks if I mind telling her what happened.

'I went on a new medication,' I tell her, 'and it made me suicidal.'

She thanks me for sharing with her, then takes a measured pause. 'I don't want this to be the Oppression Olympics,' she says. 'But we all feel that way sometimes. It's important to remember that we have an accountability to others, and to handle it with more professionalism.'

'Right,' I say. I can't remember if I apologise or not.

Pavan and I stop planning our wedding. How foolish, to have picked a date. When the would-be day of our wedding rolls around, we buy nice wine and order everything we like from the vegan Chinese restaurant on Johnston Street. We make a picnic on our bedroom floor, eat with leisure.

Vin Diesel has just released a single. It's a club banger that never goes hard. We play it over and over, imagining Vin Diesel crooning nervously about a girl he's too shy to talk to, and laugh ourselves giddy. I feel light for the first time in a long time. Outside it's raining, wet and miserable. Inside, the day stretches long and languid.

'People always say that their wedding day just flashes by,' I say. In some ways, this is better than a wedding.

We keep moving through cycle after cycle of lockdown.

At work, we have a virtual social gathering. We meet in small Zoom groups to talk about the impact of lockdown. We're given discussion questions, asked to get to know one another. I'm grouped with three people from the Sydney office, none of whom I've met before.

'I think the hardest part of lockdown,' one of them says, 'has been showing enough compassion for our co-workers in Melbourne.'

I think about quitting my job, remember that I can't afford to quit my job.

That week, by chance, I get a Teams message from a colleague.

Hey, she writes, *you don't have PMDD do you?*

I'm bamboozled. I've yet to meet anyone who knows what PMDD is, let alone is able to identify it from the sparse details I've shared. To me, her recognition seems magic or miracle. She tells me that she was just diagnosed, then sends me a link to an endocrinologist who specialises in PMDD. She's currently bulk-billing, because of the pandemic.

I didn't know anyone specialised in it, I type to the colleague.

She's the only one in Australia, I guess.

I stop everything I am doing and make an appointment through the endocrinologist's website. The waiting list is over a month long. Still, I feel a semblance of hope.

The colleague and I message on and off throughout the day, then move to text when it gets too personal. We've never met: she was hired after the lockdowns started. She tells me that she went on the pill, too, that it was horrible and she stopped straight away.

She tells me to get a referral to the psychologist the endocrinologist partners with, one who specialises in PMDD.

She's the only good one, my colleague writes.

—

When the co-worker recognises my illness and calls it by its name, I feel the euphoria of recognition, like, *Yes, I am finally seen!* We have a shared language for this. We know the clinical terms, the diagnostic criteria, the descriptions of 'fog lifting' and 'out of control'. Yet I can't help but wonder about her inner experience of PMDD. I'm left questioning the parts that are ignored, even reduced, by our shared language.

The act of naming an illness requires a tracing of the body and its parts. The illness is broken down into its biological components: uterus, menses, oestrogen, progesterone, allopregnanolone, neurosteroids, my body, my brain. My gaze is directed away from the experience of the illness and towards a biological cause and cure. I look at diagrams of hormones and receptors, each made up of its own tiny interlocking spirals. I experience the effects that this illness has on my psyche, my state of being, while simultaneously understanding it as a biological fact. While naming my illness—diagnosing it—is meant to be a tool for seeking treatment, it simultaneously highlights all the ways in which contemporary science is unable to do the work that succeeds naming: actually treating it.

Naming my illness means reckoning with its traceable facts: there is no cure, it is chronic, it will exist within me until menopause, the monster will return, will return, will return.

Naming carries permanence. I think of a stray cat who used to stop by my house a few days a week. He rubbed against my legs, meowed at me for attention. For weeks, I refused to name him: he was just a cat. When I gave in and named him, his visits became daily. He had taken up space in my mind, my home. Once named, he started to sleep at the end of my bed.

Naming is also a kind of myth. In 'On Truth and Lies in a Non-moral Sense', Friedrich Nietzsche articulates how, in order to name something, we must block out 90 per cent of the truth of the thing. He gives the example of *leaves*: a word that contains billions of different realities. The word *leaf* reduces not only each *type* of leaf, but each tangible, individual leaf, into a singular word, a singular name. This is what Nietzsche calls 'the first metaphor', the metaphor of language itself.

I begin to understand that naming an illness can be similarly reductive. When I name my illness, my experience of it is no longer solely my own, but a collective experience, a suite of signs and symptoms. Premenstrual dysphoric disorder becomes a framework of specific, nameable traits, a metaphor for the actual experience. My gnawing sense of dread when the dishes have not been done becomes the broad symptom of *irritation*. Me retreating to bed, or the floor, to give in to my bodily urge to cry becomes a categorisable *depression*. The flood of humiliation-relief that I experience once the bleeding starts becomes *symptoms alleviating upon the onset of menses*. When the breadth of my personal experience is named, it becomes simultaneously more understandable and less specific. Boundaries between what is my life—my individual and real grievances—and what is my illness start to form. The boundary between my ill-self and my well-self becomes distinct. I think in terms like *I am not myself*, though at all times I am and can only be myself.

There is a similar instinct in the people around me, specifically the people who love me, to view my non-mad self as my true self.

It's your body doing this. It's not you. You're just anxious. It's your anxiety.

In her memoir about illness and the history of women's medical treatment, *Hysteria*, Katerina Bryant writes: 'In writing circles, you are encouraged not to conflate writing and the self. You are not your writing. In chronic illness communities, you are encouraged similarly. You are not your illness. But on any given day, I feel like a strand of yarn woven with the things that make me a person.'

You are not your writing. You are not your illness.

But depending on the time of the month, I am always one of the dual selves my body demands of me. Who am I if not my body, my chemistry, my mind? Of course, like Bryant, I am more than my illness. I am a writer, I am an avid *Survivor* watcher, I am vegan, I am disorganised, I am my partner, my friends, my family, my community. And, slowly, I might become my ability to cope with this illness, too.

21.

When my virtual appointment with the endocrinologist rolls around, I take my computer to the courtyard and meet her in the sun. She explains the science behind PMDD to me, tells me that they can't really be sure of anything—there's not much money in women's health, and even the promising trials lack funding for second rounds.

I tell her that I am on the pill now, how bad it was, how I am more stable now, but always low. She tells me that, though my body may have adjusted to the constant stream of hormones, it makes sense that I'm constantly feeling low. I am taking the hormone my body hates every single day.

'Some people have adverse reactions to Yaz,' she tells me. 'It might be worth coming off it.'

The truth is that I am too scared to act. I can't go back to how I felt, how my body felt, those first two days on the pill. I tell her that I am scared of the effects of withdrawal, of another episode, and she understands. She asks me to talk her through my symptoms, my calendar of moods. I tell her about the mood swings, the depression, the combativeness, the aches behind my knee.

When I mention the knee thing she stops and raises her eyebrows.

'Is it always in the same knee?' she asks.

'I think so,' I tell her. 'The right.'

'That's it, then,' she says. 'Physical aches are usually the differentiating factor between premenstrual dysphoric disorder and a pre-existing mental illness that's been exacerbated by premenstrual symptoms.'

She gives me a referral to the psychologist who specialises in PMDD, and suggests switching to an oestrogen-only pill if I still want the contraceptive benefits.

It's around this time that Pavan and I start to fight. It's no longer a once-a-month thing but an all-the-time thing. Afterwards, I try to remember the details but come back foggy. I remember us criss-crossing St Georges Road, me in tears again. We are fighting about—something—I don't know. I am being difficult. Whatever Pavan says to cheer the mood leaves me snappy and cold.

'What would Dickie do?' he asks, desperate to see any other side of me.

I say something like *fuck you*, or perhaps I don't say anything at all. Then he says nothing at all, retreats inwards, and that makes me angry, too. In my memory, we are both inside and outside. In one version, he is mad at me. In another version, I am mad at him. At some point, he tries to grab my hand. I push him off too viciously and he says something like, *You want to hit me right now, don't you?* and I tell him that *I would never*, even though he's right. I do want to. The realisation should leave me cold and embarrassed, but I am too far gone to back down. Instead, I say something like, *How horrible do you think I am?* It's not even a trick question.

In other memories of this fight we are delirious. Laughing. We are pushing each other to manic tears, not angry tears. Perhaps he is not poking me at all, but tickling me.

Then he says, 'No one else could ever love you.'

It could be a joke, the way he says it. But, in the same way that he knows that I want to hit him, I know that he means it.

'No one else would put up with you.'

I think I have been pushing him to this point: to the point where he says something big enough to hold the anger I feel. I tell him that we need some space to break out of this fight, this dynamic, this whatever. We sleep separately. Or perhaps we only take a few hours apart. I can't remember.

My mum once said that people behave worst around those they trust the most, because they know their person won't leave. She is talking about toddlers. She is talking about how they yell and scream and cry in supermarkets because they feel safe enough to do so. But if they think their parent will actually leave, big tantrums turn to small, sniffly sobs. No longer safe, they pull themselves together. I think I am acting like a toddler. I push Pavan to the brink of leaving, only to rein myself in at the thought that he might.

In our first session, the new psychologist uses the term *vulnerable brain*. She means that I am more sensitive to stimulus: hormones, medications, changes in chemistry. I get caught in the poetics of it: defenceless against ideas, susceptible to thoughts.

At the time of my treatment, one of the newest theories of premenstrual dysphoric disorder built on the fact that, before entering the menses phase of the menstrual cycle, the body floods with progesterone. This progesterone flows through the reproductive system and beyond, and as progesterone enters the brain, it's converted to a chemical called allopregnanolone, 'allo' for short. For most people, allo has a calming effect. For those with PMDD, the brain responds differently. My psychologist describes it as an allergic reaction. Stress levels rise, irritation snowballs, emotions, including aggression, are heightened.

There are other theories, too. Some doctors believe that the body is not reacting to too much allo, but too little. Perhaps something malfunctions at the point of production or conversion, leaving the brain with too much progesterone and too little allo. Perhaps it's not the quantity at all, but a reaction to the change. My moods are responding to changes in hormone levels like a stomach lurching to the loops and dips of a rollercoaster.

When Pavan and I come back together, we are calm, though still nervous and bruised. We apologise. We hold each other. He feels shame for what he said, and I feel shame for how I acted. Even though he doesn't say it—would never say it—I feel the weight of having driven him there. This behaviour feels more me than him. I have made him culpable for my own anger.

He tells me that he didn't mean what he said, and I tell him that it's okay if he did, that two things can be true.

He can mean it and not mean it, too.

22.

My psychologist believes that hormones can shape a memory.

'It's like childbirth,' she says. 'No one would go through it a second time if they could recall the whole of the pain. Instead of dulling the pain itself, our bodies dull the memory.'

I think of how I wake up the morning of my period, blissful and oblivious to my pain from the night before. Outside of the luteal phase, I can hardly remember how distressed I was. Within the luteal phase, I can hardly remember ever being okay. I find myself severed: one self who only remembers the pain, and one self who can barely poke at its surface. I think of all the times I've tried to remember what I've done, what I'm capable of, and my recollections have appeared hazy and blurred.

This forgetting sounds mythical. It is not. Rather, forgetting feels like a shadow. The pain is gone and the shape of it is all that's left. Doubt fills in the details. Other people with premenstrual dysphoric disorder have described the end of the luteal phase as being like a cloud has lifted, or the difference between day and night, but to me neither is quite right. I never feel the fog of PMDD lift; it is more like startling upon a vague memory that it was there at all. One moment I'm prostrate on my bedroom floor, the sickest I've been in my life. The next I'm laughing in the courtyard, the sun on my face, warm with how good life is. There's no transitory self between the two. Rather, the self with sun on my face has completely forgotten about the self prostrate on the floor. The shock is in remembering.

Forgetting is a kind of horror. In werewolf lore, many werecreatures have no memory of what they have done in their lycanthropic state. They wake, surrounded by blood and covered in scratches, and have to piece together the mystery of the night before. Bruce Banner does not remember his actions as the Hulk; somehow, though, he still has to live with them. In horror films, the horror itself is often absent—the camera cuts away, and the viewer is left to imagine the carnage. In *Raw*, Justine wakes the morning after a party to find her bed covered in blood. Her friend is in the bed next to her. She tries to shake him awake, but he is still. Dead. His leg is missing, half devoured. She screams, horrified by what she might have done, until she realises the horrific act wasn't hers at all.

My forgetting is not a were-forgetting; it's not a Hulk-forgetting, either. Perhaps it's closest to Justine's: I remember what I might be capable of, and then the details are blurry. I wake in fear of what I might have done, not quite sure how horrible I felt, or how horribly I acted.

Some of the most promising research into PMDD has been done on rats.

The rats are kept in cages of two or three, with free access to food and water. The cages remain indoors, with an artificial day and an artificial night. Each morning, researchers take vaginal swabs from the female rats to determine where they are in their cycles. After two normal cycles, the rats are injected with two doses of either fluoxetine—Prozac—or a saline solution. An hour after their second dose, the rats are killed, and their brains are sampled.

Researchers found that the brains of female rats who were injected with fluoxetine contained higher levels of allopregnanolone than both the male rats and the rats injected with saline. This is promising—for humans, not for rats. It shows that fluoxetine operates not only to increase serotonin levels in the brain, but, as a lucky side effect, also operates on neurosteroids. In other words, fluoxetine could have near-immediate benefits when treating PMDD and postpartum depression. We know this to be true: while most selective serotonin reuptake inhibitors (SSRIs) take weeks, even months, to increase serotonin in the brain, fluoxetine can be an exception. People with PMDD often see their symptoms alleviated within hours of taking Prozac.

In other studies, researchers have measured the effect of allopregnanolone on the behaviour of rats and mice. When allopregnanolone levels are low in mice, they show increased levels of anxiety and depression. They are less social. They're worse at maze tests. They take less pleasure from sugar water. They're slower in forced swimming tests.

Before the lockdowns, in a creative-writing class I took, the teacher talked about how animal studies revealed our limited imaginations as humans. Too often, humans would test the social dynamics of animals by providing four sheep with three food bowls, then recording the results.

'What happens if you give four sheep five bowls?' said the teacher. 'We never think to ask.'

There are other problems with animal studies, too. The researcher's goal is not the animal's goal. When we put a rat in a maze, we assume they want to find the cheese. If they are slow, we assume they have failed. We never think to ask what the rat's goal is—if they want the cheese that day, or if they're just looking to explore the world outside their cage.

When I read these studies, I imagine myself as one of the lab rats, my functions stripped back to the least number of variables. Each morning, I wake to the same artificial light at the same predetermined time. I eat the same food, see the same one or two other rats. As my hormone levels and neurosteroids are altered, I go mad. I fail my artificial tests—I run out of the gate too quickly, start to swim too slowly. I withdraw from my peers, eat too much then too little. I can't help but wonder about the variables that aren't measured—variables that have no place in a scientific study. If these hormonal rats were let to run free, perhaps they wouldn't be so withdrawn. If these rats were able to see more than the same four walls, the same artificial lights, perhaps they wouldn't be so anxious.

I can already see how a cage can make an illness worse.

For the first few weeks, my psychologist asks me to keep track of my feelings: not only the big ones, but the small ones too. One of the most common treatments for PMDD involves building a person's ability to sit with discomfort. She asks me to sit with my feelings, acknowledge them, but not act on them. At times, I feel like I'm building a chronology of all the little things that upset me on a day-to-day basis. We have a foster dog stay with us, and it's my housemate's turn to pick up the poo. I see him throwing it all into a pile in the corner of the yard. When I tell him to throw it away properly, he looks at me like I'm an idiot.

'Where else am I supposed to put it?' he scoffs.

I suggest the bin and for a split moment I perceive on his face an expression that I take to mean he hasn't thought of this. I want to pull my hair out; it's a small discomfort.

Pavan is cooking in the kitchen. The counter is littered with ingredients—breadcrumbs, tomato guts, garlic skin—that he promises to clean up afterwards. From the couch, I see him wiping the breadcrumbs from the bench straight onto the floor. I bite my tongue, write it down, don't say anything. It's just discomfort.

By the end of the week, I want to scream and yell and tell the people I'm living with how ashamed they should feel about their domestic misdeeds. Instead, I go to the bedroom. I curl up on the floor and feel miserable. When Pavan comes to check on me, I say only that I'm not feeling so good and that I'm learning to sit with it. I tell myself that it will be fine; no one has died, nothing bad has happened. But I feel terrible, cranky, really really bad.

When I next meet with my psychologist, I tell her that I tracked the discomfort, but said nothing. I tell her how horrible it felt, and how hard it was. I half expect her to revoke her instructions, to tell me that I had a right to get angry.

'That's good,' she says. 'You don't need to feel good. You just need to not make it worse.'

I don't feel anger; I feel relief. It's okay for me to be miserable. I can at least try to not make others miserable, too.

23.

On the news, I see small groups of protestors in the city, shouting in the empty streets about Dictator Dan and lockdown restrictions. They look foolish, selfish. We haven't got a vaccine yet. They're putting lives at risk.

Despite my growing anger towards the medical system, I will not abandon it. These lockdowns are hard, but they're necessary. I think of my friends who are immunocompromised, who have to deal with hospitals, discomfort, invasive procedure after invasive procedure. I believe we can do better, but I also know that this is the best we have. To abandon science, to abandon these attempts at getting it right, feels just as misguided as to pretend that medicine can't do better, too.

The type of therapy my psychologist champions is called dialectical behaviour therapy, or DBT. In some ways, DBT mirrors cognitive behavioural therapy (CBT), where patients learn to recognise troubling thoughts and develop strategies to redirect them. But DBT expands on CBT in a few critical ways. While both incorporate mindfulness practices, DBT starts with the radical understanding that these thoughts are normal; that they will come up, and that, instead of fighting them, we must learn to live with them. Rather than teaching patients to redirect thoughts, DBT teaches us to sit with the discomfort of these thoughts, to accept them, and to build the capacity for emotional regulation required to stop troubling thoughts from escalating into troubling behaviours.

I picture the difference like this: Carrie is told that her anger is normal, is rational, is the appropriate response to a horrific situation. Someone takes her aside, tells her that yes, what you feel is monstrous, but you do not have to be the monster. Her rage is heard and disaster, just maybe, is averted.

Dialectical behaviour therapy was developed by Dr Marsha Linehan. At seventeen, Linehan was institutionalised for extreme social withdrawal. She was sent to the Institute of Living in Hartford, Connecticut, a psychiatric facility, where she was diagnosed with schizophrenia and held in total isolation. It was 1961. The hospital staff gave her a room containing only a bed, a chair and a small, barred window: nothing she could hurt herself with. Because, given the chance, Linehan would hurt herself. Prior to her admission, she had burnt herself with cigarettes and slashed at her body with anything she could find.

In my second-last year of high school, my family moved to Springthorpe, a newly developed neighbourhood in Macleod, next to the deserted Mont Park Asylum. This 'Hospital for the Insane' was opened in 1912 under the *Lunacy Act* of 1903. Here again: moons and madness. It operated until the mid-1990s.

The first time my grandpa came to visit, he told me that he used to drive his van there sometimes, for deliveries or excursions.

'Once I drove past and they were hosing them all down,' he said. 'All of them, just outside, with a hose. Like a shower or something.'

I pictured a firehose, felt a ghostly horror down my spine.

When Mont Park opened, its facilities were world-class. It was a huge, sprawling complex of red-brick buildings surrounded by trees, fields and lakes. There were rest rooms, treatment rooms, greenhouses, staff accommodation, even a gymnasium. Many patients found work on the institution's farms, or as artisans: carpenters, blacksmiths, tailors. There was a whole ecosystem within the hospital—fields, pens for cows and pigs, storerooms for fruit and vegetables—the remnants of which we later walked the family dogs through.

While in the care of the Institute of Living, Linehan was dosed with a suite of drugs that, in combination, left her numb and sedated. They performed Freudian analysis and electroshock therapy on her. After 30 sessions of electric shocks—sixteen sessions the first round, fourteen the second—nothing had changed. Linehan was sent back into isolation. With nothing to do, she banged her head against the wall and the floor, over and over again.

'I was in hell,' said Linehan in an interview with *The New York Times*. 'I made a vow: *When I get out, I'm going to come back and get others out of here.*'

In May 1963, Linehan was released from the Institute of Living. *During 26 months of hospitalisation*, her discharge statement notes, *Miss Linehan was, for a considerable part of this time, one of the most disturbed patients in the hospital.*

Without knowing what was wrong with her, the medical team at the Institute of Living were ill-equipped to help her.

By 1963—the same year that, on the other side of the world, Marsha Linehan was being released from her own asylum—the patient population of Mont Park rose to fifteen hundred. Some two hundred of them were employed within the hospital, producing food or goods for both themselves and other asylums around Melbourne. The remaining majority, who were unable to work, were often confined to their cells—wards—or overcrowded cages. Some were restrained with straitjackets or locked in padded rooms. They repeated the same routines, walked through the same halls, sat in the same small cells, day after day. According to the Springthorpe Heritage Project, a group run by local-history enthusiasts, 'Many patients under these circumstances, with an unchanging pattern day in and day out, over the passage of time, became very institutionalised, with little independent thought, apathetic, obedient, and totally reliant on the system.'

After school, my friends and I would explore the asylum. Most of the property was owned by La Trobe University, but it was deserted, cobwebbed with vines and falling plaster. We would wander through its abandoned halls during the day, drink beers on the roof at night.

It was easy to get in. There were no fences, no security. When we first moved to Macleod, most of the doors to the asylum were unlocked and had been for years. While nearly all the rooms were trashed and vandalised, with mushrooms sprouting through the floor, some contained the ghosts of an earlier time. In one room, I found a vending machine stocked with early-90s Coca-Cola cans, the word *Coke* written in a stiff serif font: antiques to a teenager in the late 2000s. We shook the machine, trying to get the bottles to fall, but failed. Another room led to the frame of a greenhouse or courtyard, its windows and ceiling smashed. The ground was overgrown, teenage saplings sprouting like weeds in the middle.

Down a hallway, we looked through barred windows into rooms padded white like marshmallows. They were locked tight. We stared, horrified, then tried a room on the opposite side of the hall. Open. The walls were lined with metal drawers and benches. In the middle of the concrete floor stood a solitary surgical bed.

'Do you think they performed lobotomies here?' my friend asked.

I opened one of the drawers. It was empty, yet my mind filled it with scalpels, pliers, long, thin picks and hammers. I wanted to leave.

Later, I asked my dad why the asylum closed. He wasn't sure. 'Probably because of medicine,' he told me. 'For a long time, people just had no idea what to do with mental illness. Many of the people who were put in Mont Park back then would probably live happy, healthy lives today.'

Later, I read that the hospital did perform lobotomies. In 1953, the neurosurgical unit was opened in Mont Park, and the following year 43 lobotomies were carried out on patients. During the operation, connections between the prefrontal cortex and the frontal lobes of the brain were physically severed. Some patients' behaviour improved, but at a cost: they could no longer control their impulses, or they became unnaturally calm, or they experienced a total absence of feeling. At the time, Mont Park was considered cutting-edge in its approach to treatment. Alongside lobotomies, it performed electroconvulsive therapies—often without anaesthetic—leaving patients with bone damage, shattered teeth and muscular tears. It also performed the newly developed insulin therapy for schizophrenia, through which patients were routinely dosed with high levels of insulin, putting them into a comatose state each day, for several weeks.

After leaving the Institute of Living, Marsha Linehan went to university. She was committed to helping what she described as the very worst cases, the 'super suicidal' people.

'I figured these are the most miserable people in the world—they think they're evil, that they're bad, bad, bad—and I understood that they weren't,' she said. 'I understood their suffering because I'd been there, in hell, with no idea how to get out.'

In 1993, the year I was born, Marsha Linehan made good on her vow. She published an article in the *American Journal of Psychotherapy*, outlining the success of her early trials of dialectical behaviour therapy. In her article, she proposes a theoretic framework for DBT, outlining both its challenges and successes. She writes about how a therapist's mind must 'dance with movement, speed and flow', and how a therapist must have the humility to radically accept a patient's distress, without reducing it. There is no singular way to treat a person who is distressed, suicidal, feeling monstrous. She outlines acceptance skills not as a pathway to change, but as a pathway to making life more liveable.

When my psychologist tells me Dr Marsha Linehan's story, she mentions that DBT was originally developed for people with borderline personality disorder. Supposedly, Linehan began her research by flicking through the DSM, looking for the best fit. She wanted to help people who were seriously unwell, but to get any funding, she needed a diagnosis. So, she picked BPD.

In therapy, borderline patients are known to be monstrous—manipulative, hostile, notorious for storming out of sessions or threatening suicide. By accepting them at their worst, Linehan found that patients were more likely to stay. And a patient who will stay is easier to treat than a patient who won't. There is tension in accepting the bad. It feels wrong to reinforce the duality of selves that unwell people experience. It feels wrong to accept the monstrous identities they have built for themselves. But when Linehan listened to their monstrous thoughts, she could accept that in light of all this pain—this emptiness, this rage—all the cutting and burning and gashing begins to make sense.

The Institute of Living is still operational today. It has a page on its website dedicated to dialectical behaviour therapy. There I read a quote from Linehan: 'The overall goal of DBT skills training is to help you increase your resilience and build a life experienced as worth living.' There is no mention of her time within the walls of the facility.

24.

I make another virtual appointment with my GP. The whole week leading up, I dread it. I don't want to talk to her. My bra is the wrong size, my shirt feels stiff. I am perpetually uncomfortable.

I don't want to go on SSRIs, and then I do. I am still on the pill, still Yaz, still too scared to go off it, even though the stability it brings means I constantly feel low. I can tell that I am not okay; still, I can't shake my fear of trying yet another new medication. I read stories online of people having good experiences with Prozac, and bad ones, too. *Amped up my suicidal thoughts*, one person writes. *Absolutely saved my life*, writes another.

My endocrinologist reminds me that medical research is decades behind where it could be when it comes to premenstrual dysphoric disorder. She tells me that there has been one clinical trial for a drug that targets PMDD directly, but that any viable medication is still years away. Until then, the options are limited: SSRIs, the pill, medical menopause. Without medicine to treat this illness specifically, I am subject to the side effects of other medications. I remember how, when I was little, my mother told me that there was no such thing as a side effect, not really.

'They're all just effects of the medication,' she said. 'We just give effects we don't want a different name.'

I flip the script around in my head. The pill: medication to make you depressed. Side effect: you won't get pregnant. Prozac: a pill to kill your sex life. Side effect: you might be happy.

When the time comes to call my doctor, I make an excuse and push the appointment back. I tell myself that I am feeling okay, that I am better now, that two weeks off work was good enough.

I'm scared that change will make this worse—more scared than I am of acknowledging that avoiding change means not making it better. I try to refocus on small and simple habits to make the dark thoughts fade away: I start walking again, doing yoga, journalling.

I watch organising videos on YouTube. I start making lists. I return to my articles on resilience. I try to embrace motivational quotes. I want to learn how to carry this weight on my own. Since going on the pill I have been constantly cranky, but I'm breathing through it.

When I cook dinner, Pavan turns his nose up at one of the ingredients and I want to cry, but I don't. I write it down in my journal and call it progress. When I ask Pavan to help clean, he jokes that I am better at it anyway. I want to scream; I am not good at it, not good at any of this, but I am doing it anyway. My thread is pulled taut. I breathe. I'm surprised when I do not snap.

—

By October 2020, it's official: Melbourne has had the longest continuous lockdown in the world. From the inside, it feels rhythmic. The smallest changes to the rules make the world crack open, or snap shut.

I feel completely empty inside. Despite my best efforts, I'm back to staring at walls, lacking the motivation to do anything. I am getting better at sitting with discomfort, but that's all there is: sitting with it.

My work routine is shattered. Some days I am so dramatic; I think to myself, *I would rather die than work today*, then I work anyway. I get hardly anything done. In a good week, I finish 90 per cent of a new website. I wake up at 5.30 a.m., too anxious to sleep, and work instead. Late on Friday, my boss calls to say that the project's off.

'But you did a good job,' she adds, as a hopeful aside.

I remind myself that if I didn't go back to work, I couldn't afford the new therapist. I remind myself that I don't want to die, I just want the time to pass.

Pavan's only remaining hobby is cooking. If he didn't cook, I wouldn't eat. I barely have an appetite. I don't do much to take care of myself, either. I rarely shower, wear the same clothes for days on end. No one notices.

Towards the end of the Stage 4 lockdown, though we don't know it's the end, I bend the rules. I leave my house to sit on a friend's front lawn. I meet the friend's housemate and realise that they are the first new person I have met in nearly ten months.

For the first time since the lockdowns started, I get to hear details of someone new's life. They tell me about their girlfriend, what they do for work. We talk about editing, art, writing, and even though the conversation is hardly revolutionary, it fills me with something new. I leave feeling inspired. When I get home, I write for the first time in months.

I call my boss and try to work with her on my feelings about work. I want to make it better, but I don't know how.

'I feel like I'm underperforming,' I say, 'but when I try to find a framework to measure my performance against, there is none. I don't know what I should be working on, what I should prioritise. I feel like as soon as I finish something it's not wanted anymore.'

'Well, you are underperforming,' says my boss. 'You need to communicate with me what you need, or I can't do anything.'

It feels fair, but I end the call deflated.

The truth is that I don't know what to ask for. For projects not to be cancelled. For the world to stop spinning. For it to go back to how it was before. I beat myself up about my own laziness, about how the two weeks off work only dragged me deeper into the vortex, not out.

By late October, restrictions start to ease again. We're allowed to sit in the park, we can move freely during our morning walks. The pub across the street even reopens, with limited outdoor-only capacity.

We meet some friends in Edinburgh Gardens, bring snacks and drinks. The park is packed: everyone has the same idea. We sit and talk and laugh, but no one has much to say. I find myself wanting to leave early, go home with Pavan and just cuddle up in front of the TV instead. I feel sullen and boring, like I've forgotten how to have a good time.

When we get home, Pavan and I talk about friendship.

'I feel like there are two stages of friendships,' Pavan says. 'The stage where you make memories together, and the stage where you sit around and catch up.'

We decide that we need to make memories for a bit. We need to do the things we want to talk about.

On a Tuesday, I hand in my four weeks' notice. I have no back-up plan, no idea how I will make money. The only certainty I feel is that I can't do it anymore.

I meet with my boss, and her boss. They both seem saddened by the news, though they meet it without resistance. They ask me to write my handover notes and finish up by the end of the week. They'll pay the rest of my notice period out. There is no exit interview. I try to send a goodbye email at 4 p.m. on my final day, but I'm already off the system.

25.

Pavan keeps telling me that we're fine for money, but I know he's stressed, too. From the age of fourteen and three-quarters, I've had a job, and been squirrelling away my pay for some unknown future. I know that I'm lucky: I now have enough in my bank account to get me through three months without work—more with Pavan's help—but I can't make myself feel safe.

Certain facts roll through my mind: that women retire with less super than men, that career breaks for the caring duties that inevitably become their burden leave women worse off, that too many women rely on their partners and families, that senior women belong to one of the lowest earning income groups in Australia and are the fastest growing cohort of people experiencing homelessness. My anxiety is not misplaced, even if the danger is not imminent. The reality is that there is still a part of me that believes that I am no good, that I'll never work again.

Without work, my days become unsettlingly calm. I waste the extra time. I try to write, then end up downloading *The Sims*: a game

I played in high school. I grow bored within an hour but keep playing anyway.

Across from me, Pavan is between scripts. He's working on a song, headphones on. He's bobbing up and down, singing; he's been doing it for days. He can go for hours at a time. I try to write but I come up short. I'm no longer measuring myself against the work—I'm measuring myself against him. How long he can sit at a desk, how long he can work on his art.

At night, I struggle to sleep. Pavan stays up late, making music. When he comes to bed, I am barely asleep and am irritated about being woken. He kicks and squirms until I tell him to stop, but even the stopping doesn't help. I can feel him next to me, uncomfortable and awake, trying desperately not to disturb me.

'I don't mean to fidget,' he says.

I remember other nights, where he would kick and squirm and I'd pull him close, ask to be the big spoon, not let it bother me.

Now, I feel angry because I am tired. I feel angry because I thought that quitting work would make me a nicer person to be around. I am not happy. I am still defective, wrong. I have everything I need, and yet my stomach contorts with grief. I want to do the right thing, and I don't think it's right to put someone else through this trouble, too.

In her book *The Curse*, Karen Houppert gives voice to the numerous ways in which menstruation has been stigmatised across millennia of Western culture. She argues that the real trial of menstruation is not hormones, or PMS, or cramps, but the shame that surrounds it: 'The mostly male-dominated media have set a tone that shapes women's experiences for them, defining what they are allowed to feel about their periods, their bodies, and their sexuality.' According to her, it's through our culture of sexism that 'confident girls learn to be self-conscious teens'.

While reading her book, I am spun once more through a duality of selves. I try to remind myself how two things can be true. A period can be normal, animal, uneventful. It can also be a rotten, nasty thing.

I read more testimonies of women who have experienced PMDD, how they are driven mad by housework, how they become bad partners, how they cry and scream and yell. In all the stories, Houppert narrows in on the ways these women are struggling—really struggling—and how they turn not to the sexist burdens placed on them to explain this struggle, but to PMS.

One of the women Houppert interviewed, like many women, only developed PMS symptoms after having children. Her moods were destroying her relationship. She lost patience, yelled at her husband, yelled at the kids. More than anything, she feared losing control. Her husband, a physician, asked her to try Prozac. At first, she was reluctant. She didn't want to become a Stepford wife. When she finally relented, she felt better almost overnight.

'My husband was thrilled,' she tells Houppert.

Her story reads as dystopia: a woman needs help, doesn't get help, and is instead medicated by a man to make her more docile and to stop her requests for help. When Houppert asks her to recall why her PMS symptoms were so frightening to her, she struggles to answer.

'I was flying off the handle, overreacting,' she says. 'It seems like the rest of the world is wrong, and if they'd only listen to you, they'd realise.'

Through these stories, Houppert suggests that, rather than being driven mad by PMDD, these women are experiencing a rational level of anger in response to an unfair world. It is not these women who are the problem, but the culture that surrounds them.

My own duality of selves can be blinding. Just because my well-self can tolerate discomfort, doesn't mean that my ill-self is wrong to be upset. I worry that I am still writing myself into the sexist dystopia that Houppert tries to warn against. At the same time, I can see that by staying on the pill, by not taking the Prozac, I am making everyone else miserable, too. I feel like an army ant, walking death spirals around the question of whether it's me who is sick, or the world.

I remind myself again that two things can be true.

There are days when I don't think I can do this anymore. Any of it: trying to write, living with a man, living at all. My doctor describes my symptoms as burnout, but I'm doing less than ever. The women I worked with ran laps around me. Now, I'm barely even writing. Other women have children, families, responsibilities; I'm in tears over a couple of dishes left in the sink each night and an unmade bed each morning.

There are days when I want to scream at Pavan—just put the toilet paper back on the roll, *please!* Please, just one little act of care for me. But I'm supposed to be sitting with discomfort, not acting on it. It's not worth fighting over the small stuff. I'm jealous of Pavan's ability to not care if the dishes aren't done, the bin's overflowing, the bed's unmade and there are clothes on the floor. Then my thinking flips: compared to some, I have a high tolerance for grot. I'm fine with dishes left overnight, just not for days. I can go weeks without doing laundry. I do not want to talk about how infrequently I change my sheets. There is no regularity to my vacuuming. I am not a neat freak, yet every partner I have been with has made me feel like one.

Somewhere around this time, I read Jenny Offill's *Dept. of Speculation* and am struck by the notion of art monsters. Offill writes: 'My plan was never to get married. I was going to be an art monster instead. Women almost never become art monsters because art monsters only concern themselves with art, never mundane things. Nabokov didn't even fold his own umbrella. Vera licked his stamps for him.' I feel that I am licking too many stamps for Pavan. I am desperate for him to lick a stamp for me.

'Do you realise,' I ask Pavan, dripping with snot and tears, 'that when *you* don't do it, I feel like you're just assuming that I will?'

'That's not true,' he says.

'If you use the last piece of toilet paper, who is going to replace it?'

'I will,' he says. 'Later.'

I give him a baffled look. I need more hands than I possess to count the occasions on which he's called me from the toilet, stuck and panicked.

'And when you don't? How does it magically get replaced?'

He shakes his head. 'You're not getting me. I don't expect you to do it—I will do it, just later.'

I want to slam my head into a wall, swallow my fist, drive a car into a tree. 'But *you* don't do it later. *I* do it later.'

He says that he knows, but that's not how it's supposed to be. 'I really, really believe that I'm going to do it later,' he says. 'I just forget sometimes.'

'So don't leave it until later.' I sound manic, haggard, deranged. 'If you know you forget, then do better. Do it *now*.'

'I'm trying,' Pavan says.

The worst part is that I believe him. It's a hopeless realisation. I have all these negative thoughts, like: *This man isn't maliciously incompetent, he's just incompetent.* I imagine having this feeling for the rest of my life. Always being the one to clean the bathroom. Always replacing the toilet roll. Always taking the bins out. Always doing the laundry. My head feels full to bursting. I can't think.

There are days when I wish I could cope with all of this, and days when I wish I didn't have to. The burden of building tolerance feels unfair. I'm reminded of a scene in *Raw* where Justine wobbles across campus, wearing too-big heels forced on her by an older college student. How much discomfort women have already been taught to bear.

The morning after a particularly terrible night, Pavan comes to me with a plan.

'We need separate workspaces,' he says. Since leaving my job, we've been trying to work on our art side by side. He shifts around, stomps his feet, dances. I get cranky, tell him that he's being distracting, when really I'm distracted anyway. He suggests moving his desk to the upstairs room, and the bed downstairs, where I can write, too. It makes sense. He is working more than I am, and later into the night, too. It would give us both some space.

'Unless you have an alternative, of course,' he says.

For some reason, I start crying.

'We're not breaking up,' he says.

I tell him I know. I tell him that I don't mean to cry.

'I'm going to get out of the house for a little while,' I say. 'I don't want to cry in front of you—it makes things confusing—I just need to figure out what I actually think.'

I take my notebook to the pub, order a glass of house red and sit outside with it. The weather is warm: it almost feels like summer is here.

I sit there for hours, trying to figure out why I am upset, if I am upset at all. I jot down thought after thought, trying to write my way to understanding.

By the end of it I realise that it's not about him; it's not about whether we're growing apart or fighting too much. I don't feel anxious about him asking for space. It's about me. It's about me wanting to be okay enough to make art again. It's about the fact that I'm jealous of his ability to do things—to function—to forget about the world and just create. I think that he is more deserving of his own room in which to do this—he will use it better, more productively—but I want to deserve that space too. I know he's making the right decision by separating our workspaces. I can't keep pretending to write in the same room as him, comparing myself to him, and I am devastated that I have come to this. I want to write a story of my life where I can work, where I can function, where I can be happy. But I still feel myself spiralling in all the wrong directions. I'm upset because if I give him what he is asking for—space for him to work and make art—I feel that I will be putting myself back at square one: moving between my bed and my desk, with just the same four walls around me, still mad, still depressed, still a little bit hysterical.

When I get back home, Pavan has already moved the furniture. The bed and my small desk are downstairs, his huge desk in pieces upstairs. The top of that desk is too big for me to hold, let alone move up a flight of stairs. I don't know how he carried it alone.

'I think I got so upset,' I start, 'because I know that you deserve your own space to work, but I want to deserve it, too.'

'I don't follow,' he says. 'Us in the same space just isn't working anymore.'

'I know it's not working,' I say. 'I don't really know what I'm asking for—just that I think it will be bad for me to be stuck in the same room again. I think I want a space of my own. I want to feel like I deserve it.'

'You want the upstairs room?' he asks.

It's unspeakably hard for me to say yes. But I say it.

I expect him to be angry, or annoyed. I feel that I am asking too much.

'Okay,' is all he says. He doesn't look mad or disappointed or like it's any burden at all. 'Will you help me move my desk back?'

26.

I tell my psychologist that, even without work, I'm no better. She asks me about the pill, if I'm still on it, how it's going.

'It's fine,' I say. I'm sullen. 'My mood is stable.'

'Do you think it might be stable but . . . low stable?' she hedges.

'Yes,' I say, then think for a moment. 'I've thought about going off it, but I'm scared about how bad it was to go on it in the first place. I don't want to get that bad again. I don't know if I can take it. I don't know if Pavan can take it.'

She says that maybe I don't have to come off it.

'You know, fluoxetine—Prozac—can be really effective.'

I set up my study upstairs. I have the whole room to myself, and just a desk in it. I fill the space with plants, burn incense on the windowsill. I can hear Pavan's music through the floorboards and it makes me feel close to him. I don't get much writing done, but I try. For the first time in a long time, I don't feel shame about how much I get done, or don't get done.

Outside, time continues to move forward. It's hard to leave the house, but I know that I need to. I meet an ex-manager for a drink in Preston—a boss from before my old boss. He's a 40-year-old man with a dog named after a type of pasta. I tell him I've quit and he takes the news like he's been expecting it for a while.

'That place is toxic,' he says. 'I'm stoked you're out.'

He tells me about a job that's going at his new workplace. Government, internal communications. He's about to quit too, move away from the city, maybe buy a house, have a family, all of that stuff.

'You could really help them out,' he says.

'I don't know,' I say. 'I was pretty rubbish by the end there.'

'Nah. It'll be easy for you. I'll be your reference, if you're worried.'

I'm grateful, relieved. I tell him that I'll apply, and we get another round. We bitch and moan about my old job. He swears the new workplace is better.

After a few weeks, an old client from my very first workplace emails me, looking for a copywriter—freelance. The job pays more than I've been paid in a long time. They tell me that they remember me from way back—years ago now—and couldn't think of anyone better for their new project.

I take the flattery to heart. I need every bit of it. Slowly, with my own space and kind words, I am able to write a story for myself in which I am deserving of things. I am writing a story in which I am not the monster.

When I tell my GP that I am ready to go on Prozac, she is relieved. I don't mention the side effects I fear: she already knows I fear them.

It doesn't matter that—even through the worst of my moods—my sex life remained wonderful. I need to be better, and this is the next stage of my plan. It's been more than six months since I started this treatment process. I've had my IUD out, tracked a baseline, gone on the pill. Now I need to move on to the next step: SSRIs.

Around the time of my initial PMDD diagnosis, in 2015, a study was conducted in which women were given a drug to block the conversion of progesterone into allopregnanolone during the luteal phase of the menstrual cycle. Thirty-two participants were chosen for the study—sixteen with PMDD and sixteen without. In comparison, trials for erectile-dysfunction medications have thousands of participants.

'There's not much money in women's medicine,' my psychologist reminds me. She says that they didn't pick the participants very well, either. 'They need to be testing women who are really unwell,' she says. 'The sample size was small. They need to be sure that the women they are testing really have PMDD and not another menstruation-related mood disorder.'

While the results of the trial were promising, little came of it. It might even have delayed more comprehensive research into the illness, which is only now gaining some momentum. Fluoxetine, one of the first SSRIs developed, works by slowing the brain's reabsorption of serotonin to allow a reserve to build up. It can take months before the cumulative effect is noticed. But for people with PMDD, fluoxetine is not experienced like a regular SSRI. Instead of months, the effects of fluoxetine are often felt within 36 hours. It's believed that Prozac, like the drug in the 2015 study, impacts the conversion of progesterone into allo, too.

I start taking Prozac, and by the next day my dysphoria has vanished. It feels closer to magic than medicine.

I've heard that a belief in recovery alone can be enough to heal the body. Taking a placebo medication can also improve symptoms for all kinds of illnesses—mental illness, burns, cancer. A placebo won't heal burns or eliminate tumours, but it can have a positive effect on the experience of an illness, improving the way a body processes pain, or reducing the side effects caused by medications.

At times, I want to believe that I am faking it, that this illness is make-believe, because it offers me an easy pathway out: stop believing in the illness and it no longer exists. Or, alternatively, I might put all my belief into a little pill and watch the illness drift away. But just because a placebo works, doesn't mean that the illness isn't real. And just because an illness has no obvious cause, no clear-cut grounding in the reality of the body, doesn't mean that the effects of it aren't real. I think of other cultural illnesses—wind attacks, stolen genitals, lizards under the skin—and how real the experience of these illnesses must also feel.

There is a chance that Prozac had a placebo effect on me. If the science behind PMDD is not legitimate—if this medication is *not*, in fact, influencing the conversion of progesterone to allopregnanolone in my brain—then the sudden uptick in mood I experience must be due to something else. It's too soon for me to feel the true effects of the SSRI, which, as noted, can take months to become apparent. I remember Sandie Craddock, how high doses of progesterone made her calm, while the smallest doses took me to the edge. I cannot explain this difference biologically.

Fluoxetine first received FDA approval in 1987. Eli Lily, the pharmaceutical company that had invented Prozac over a decade before it was approved for humans use, developed the formula based on the theory that depression—an often stigmatised and misunderstood illness—was actually tied to chemical deficits in the brain. They began designing and testing different compounds, many based off antihistamines, to see whether they could selectively alter how serotonin was metabolised. Like other antidepressants of the era, fluoxetine was first tested on rats and dogs, then men. When I read this, my thinking becomes distorted. I think about how I am taking a drug designed for men to treat my women's issues. I am taking a drug tested on dogs to make me a little bit less of a bitch. When I think about how many rat brains were dissected and studied to develop this compound, I think perhaps these drugs are not even made for humans at all.

When I am unwell, I feel more animal—prone to acting instinctively, to lashing out and biting from fear. The drugs I take are not designed for women. But they have a happy consequence. When I take my little rat pills, my animal tension dissipates.

At first, it is also too soon to feel the side effects.

—

The difference for me between being on Prozac and being off it is night and day, ill-self and well-self. Hours after I take my first pill, I am joking and laughing. My anxiety fades. I am no longer wearing small irritations—I hardly feel them.

Pavan notices the change immediately. He doesn't say the thing I'm sure he's thinking: *You're you again.* He is just happy for me, happy with me. We cook dinner together, then eat it outside, talking about movies, about art.

'This feels like it used to feel,' I say. 'When we were house-sitting, chatting in courtyards.'

We talk about the old days, before lockdown, how we've changed. We tell ourselves stories, and I sense millions of new lives opening up before us, should we choose to live them.

27.

Within a few weeks, I move from being jobless to having two jobs. Within a few weeks, I move from unwell to well.

The job my ex-manager set me up with is in government, so the orientation is arduous. I work my way through the different training, files, documents as swiftly as I can. At lunch, I message my supervisor to tell her I'm taking a break. She laughs, tells me that I don't need to message her when I'm taking lunch. I tell her it's a hang-up from the last place I worked.

I mean, you can tell me if you want. But if I message you at lunchtime and you don't respond . . . I'm gonna assume it's because you're at lunch lol.

The smallest things bring me joy.

By the end of the day, I still haven't finished the orientation. I've drafted a staff newsletter, but nothing more. I feel that old pang of guilt: I'm not fit for work. I can't do it all. I send my supervisor an end-of-day update, even though she might laugh.

Wow, she messages back. *I hadn't expected you to get that far today.*

—

At midday on my second day, I feel myself growing drowsy. I can hardly keep my eyes open. My head starts to droop at my desk. I jolt upright, only to start drooping again.

I drink energy drinks to break the loop. It works well enough, gets me through the day. Still, I fear that I am about to lose everything—that any more side effects will break the delicate balance I am maintaining, the balance that is allowing me to piece my life together.

After work, I read through my medication pamphlet. One of the side effects is insomnia, so I've been taking it in the morning. But I am learning to understand my body. I am getting better at noticing.

I switch to taking Prozac in the evening. The term *vulnerable brain* echoes through my mind. I am small, these doses are taken by men twice my size, I have a *vulnerable brain*. I am gentle with myself. I talk to my GP, ask to lower my dose. She worries that a dose so small won't have much effect.

'SSRIs take a while to build up in the system,' she says. 'Your body just needs time to adjust.'

I tell her that I am learning to listen to my body now, and I'm not fucking around. I lower my dose.

When I am no longer sick, I am able to seek out treatment, take it seriously, advocate for myself. It's only when I am well that I can begin to heal. I used to think that resilience was something only some people had, and that I was not one of those people. My mind reacted abnormally to the regular flux of the world. I thought it was me that was lacking. After only a few weeks on Prozac, I realise that I was wrong. There is nothing innate about resilience. Depending on your circumstances, it is either there, or it is not.

My mum tells me about a hypnotist she saw once. She says my brother went, too, that the hypnotist helped him stop biting his nails. I ask her why she went.

'Sorry, it's a little ridiculous,' she says, before admitting that she went to try to stop apologising so much. It's not the best recommendation, but I go to see the hypnotherapist anyway, because I am desperately clinging to this new thread of life. I've stopped believing that only one thing can help.

In *The Body Keeps the Score*, Bessel van der Kolk writes about how 'New Age' treatments—he cites as an example eye movement desensitisation, which involves undergoing therapy while your eyes follow the therapist's fingers—have had outstanding results.

'We don't know why or how they work,' he writes. 'But they do. And we're only just starting to figure out why and how antidepressants work now, more than forty years after their conception.'

Why something works seems less important than the fact that it works.

I ride my bike to the hypnotherapist's office on a sunny January morning. She's located in Brunswick and looks the part. When I meet her, she's wearing a blue jumpsuit and colourful dangly earrings. Her hair is neat, her face unmade-up. She looks like a woman who keeps hens in her backyard, cycles her kids to kinder, visits the CERES farmers' market on weekends. She welcomes me into her office, lets me take a seat. For a while, we just talk.

'It sounds like you're being really hard on yourself,' she says.

'Yes,' I say. 'I suppose I am.'

On my second visit, the hypnotherapist asks me to tap certain points of my body rhythmically, while saying, 'Even though I'm not as funny as Pavan, I am still worthy of love.' I am embarrassed by this whole process. I am embarrassed because phrases like *worthy of love* have always felt a little naff to me, then I realise that I am embarrassed because it feels true, too. I am jealous of Pavan. I am jealous of his resilience, his happiness, his ability to believe in himself even in bad times. She tells me not to judge, just to say the words and tap.

Even though I am not as funny, even though I am not as strong, even though I am not as healthy.

I tap my forehead, my cheek, my chin, my neck, repeating these words. My eyes well with something like sadness, something like relief. I tap and repeat, tap and repeat. My throat locks. I tap against it.

Even though, even though, even though.

'Remember,' she says, 'the thing itself doesn't matter. It's what you value about it.'

Pavan is funny because he is smart, surprising, in tune, quick, clever, confident, can read a room. The hypnotherapist looks at me kindly and asks me to think about how much I value these qualities, how I love these qualities in Pavan, and I do.

'Sometimes,' she says, tapping her right brow and nodding for me to repeat after her, 'I feel jealous, because I also want to be quick, surprising, clever and confident.'

I echo her words, my voice cracking.

She nods at me knowingly. 'It's something, isn't it?'

On the bike ride home, I realise that I am still crying. I stop, pull my bike to the side and lie on the grass. My cheeks ache. My breath feels deep and whole. I don't know how to describe the feeling, only that the world is spinning, and I'm grateful to be spinning, too.

28.

For most of summer, we have zero new cases across the state. For a while, we are free. I feel happy, healthy, euphoric. Around us, the world is still falling apart. Pavan and I go out dancing and it feels like a beginning.

On Prozac, I feel well enough to do most things. I am still bruised, still sore from the year, but in the usual ways. No one emerged from the lockdowns unscathed. Some of my friendships fall back into their old patterns, others dissolve. I don't know whether it's because of me, or because of the world.

I stop asking myself those questions.

One sun-filled afternoon, a former work colleague—the one who messaged me on Teams about PMDD—and I make good on an almost-forgotten plan to catch up. She's shorter than I expected, and she says the same about me. We get too drunk and smoke cigarettes out the back of Monty's Bar. We talk about PMDD, share our strategies. I tell her how much better I am, how good Prozac is.

'I'm about to try it,' she says. 'Did it fuck up your sex life?'

I try to think. It's been a few months on Prozac, possibly a few months without sex, too.

'I'm not sure,' I say. 'It could just be a lull. Lockdown, you know.'

I try to remember how my body used to feel. Perhaps I'm doing it again: forgetting to notice.

I ask her how she is, and she tells me that it's been hard, that she has endometriosis, too.

'The treatments are basically the opposite,' she says. 'They wanted to put me on the pill to treat the endo, but I know it will make the PMDD crazy. My doctor is obsessed with fixing the physical pain first. I keep trying to tell her that I can live with one pain, I can't live with the other.'

I cringe. I remember how I felt those first few days on the pill, my abnormal reaction to a normal medication. I feel like we are whispering in dark corridors, sharing secret experiences that should not be true, yet are true. I can't imagine having endometriosis, too. I can't imagine the physical pain tangled with the psychological. I think of how, only a decade ago, no one would be trying to treat the endometriosis, either. Perhaps, in another decade, there will be more to hope for.

I get home drunk and messy, try to pull Pavan into bed. My body feels foreign to me. I feel myself getting turned on, but there's no wetness, no pleasure: just a stiff, dry pain. We start making out, but I'm too dry, too tight. He's scared I'll hurt him.

'We should buy some lube,' I slur.

'There's no rush,' he says.

In the morning, I google my symptoms and the term that pops up is *vaginal atrophy.* It's a symptom of menopause. Only months ago, I had believed that I would be depressed until menopause. I feel haunted. I can't help but laugh.

There are no new cases, until there are. Towards the end of summer, three COVID-19 cases emerge from hotel quarantine, and a third lockdown is announced. It's a snap lockdown, only five days this time. We cancel plans, stock up on groceries. On the news, the first Australians are getting the vaccine—elderly and immunocompromised people. There is a ferociousness with which I approach this lockdown. I feel like if we get this moment right, the other lockdowns will have been worth it.

We walk through Edinburgh Gardens the night before the restrictions kick in. The park is packed, like there's a festival on. Groups of teenagers are dancing under the streetlights, playing music on their phones. The rubbish bins are overflowing. Across the path, a girl squeals as her high heels get stuck in the grass. Her friends catch her, giggling, and pull her out.

I think I should be mad at them, meeting in such big groups the night before a lockdown, but I'm not. They're all young, either in high school or just out. I remember the delirium I felt during the early lockdown breaks, how we rubbed up against the limits of the law out of pure desperation. I know it's not right, but I don't know if I could have done any better at their age.

I think that—even if it's dumb and selfish and irresponsible—they need a little joy right now.

I don't know it yet, but after those first three lockdowns there will be a fourth, and a fifth, and eventually a sixth.

In her essay 'The Disordered Self', writer and doctor Marlene Benjamin writes, 'Mental illness, as stigmatised, signals to most people the farthest we can go from our humanness, from what makes us humans rather than mere animals.'

I am both drawn to and repulsed by the metaphors of illness: metaphors that turn madness into beasts and monsters. The stigma that surrounds mental illness often lingers at the edge of what we can see or make sense of. Mental illness can't be measured or touched, leaving room for doubt and fantasy. The invisible ceases to be real and more readily gives way to metaphor instead. When my illness is physical, biological, hormonal, it is somehow more *real*, more *manageable*, less susceptible to metaphor and fancy. Before the clinical lens of medicine could explain this illness for me, I wondered whether I was making the whole thing up, whether I was just a little worse at dealing with the world than other people were.

Experiencing the worst of my illness during the worst of the lockdowns drew my madness into sharp focus. It became too unbearable to ignore, and so I was finally able to seek the treatment I needed. Instead of giving in to anger about the enforced isolation, perhaps I should be grateful for what it gave me.

For Marlene Benjamin, short stays in locked hospital wards were what kept her alive during the worst of her psychotic breaks. While being discharged from one such stay, she recognised a woman being wheeled into the facility she herself was about to leave. The woman, she realised, had been discharged a few days after her own arrival—and now she was back.

'I went white, and the nurse murmured to me "Take your meds; take your meds,"' she writes. 'But it's far more problematic than just taking your meds, which are themselves often the cause of debilitating side effects and can complicate the underlying illness.'

Stigma has haunted mental illness for millennia. I have wondered whether it's this stigma that kept me from *taking my meds* for so long. With my new sense of focus, I am beginning to understand my body and its complexities. It feels unfair to subject myself to constant medication and endless side effects, to treat an illness that only plagues me some of the time.

I trust medicine. I trust my doctors. At times, I have trusted them more than I have trusted my own experience and my own body. I have lived with—I have been—my body for three decades now. When I first felt the pill's tidal effect on me, I should have trusted myself and stopped taking it. Instead, I chose to see myself as an irrational, mushy, unwieldy variable. I chose to stay on the drugs that were making my illness worse. I don't want to make the same mistake twice.

When I lower my dose of Prozac, the side effects do not go away. My dysphoria is gone, but sex remains impossible. A friend suggests that I am just not being creative enough, but the loss is absolute. I have no sex drive. Any gesture my body gives towards desire brings no pleasure, only pain.

I tell my psychologist about the side effects of Prozac, and how I feel sexless, finally castrated as Freud had presumed all along. She reminds me of my *vulnerable brain* and says that, often, medications are felt more strongly by people with PMDD.

I read and read, looking for signs that a new drug will come out—one that isn't an SSRI, one that won't shut my body down—but the world moves slowly. I read articles about anti-vaxxers and think something like *take your meds, take your meds*, but I understand their anxiety better now, too. I understand how a body can act abnormally in the face of medication, and how sometimes the best options we have feel not good enough.

For a while, I stop taking the Prozac altogether, to give my body a break, but the effects don't fade. Then I take only the smallest amounts, only during the worst of the illness, and still come out neutered. My doctor tells me that these prolonged side effects are impossible: it should be out of my body by now. I'm through with ignoring the reality in front of me.

When I run out of sessions with my psychologist and need a new referral to get more, I make an appointment not with my GP, but with the doctor who removed my IUD. I feel strange making this decision, because my GP is not a bad doctor, but I want better than good enough. I tell the new doctor what my body feels, how the Prozac is still affecting me. I tell her that I know it shouldn't be possible, that I know I could be making it all up, that none of this makes sense, but this is what is happening, and I feel it.

She tells me to slow down. 'First things first: I like to start by believing in my patient's symptoms.'

29.

There is a short story by Ali Smith that I love, called 'True Short Story'. In it, Smith records a discussion she overhears between two men about the difference between novels and short stories. The short story is a nymph, one man says, while the novel has grown into a 'flabby old whore'. Smith is fascinated by this strange literary imagining, twists it over and around in her head. She reimagines the tale of Echo, a nymph who used her jokes and stories to distract the goddess Juno from the fact that her nymph friends were slacking off. When Juno finds out, she curses Echo to only ever repeat the last words spoken by others:

> That's you sorted, Juno said.
> You sordid, Echo said.
> Right. I'm off back to the hunt, Juno said.
> The cunt, Echo said.

In Smith's telling of the story, there is room for small rebellions. I am looking for ways to reimagine my own curse, too. To look at monstrosity as something powerful, to view illness as illuminating. Like

Echo, I want to take the rotten hand I've been dealt and turn it into something new, playful, revelatory. I imagine alternative universes in which I can laugh at all of this: perhaps I am Dickie, skateboarding behind a car, not sweating the small stuff. I imagine a universe in which the side effects of medication are absurd: a non-hormonal birth control makes me attractive to rats. I imagine that I am cured with hot baths and nineteenth-century vibrators, until my skin softens and I shed it like a snake, emerging whole and new.

Somewhere between the lockdowns, I resume making plans to move to Vegas. I know that Pavan won't be coming with me. I meet this with something close to the openness we shared a year earlier, in the summer we first got together. I believe that we will be okay. I know that I will be okay, even if we're not. I feel like I am following a stranger's path—a dream from some other me, before the lockdowns—but I want to shed the skin of the past year. I am disorganised and haphazard with my planning, but I am ready for a change.

The week before I leave, Julie the marriage celebrant calls.

'You've already paid the deposit,' she says. 'Are you ever getting married?'

I tell her that I'm leaving in a week, that the world isn't conspiring for us to get married, that it was a nice idea, but it's not going to happen.

She says: 'I can do a wedding in a week.'

I tell her we'll think about it, and hang up. We're in the park, with coffees, walking spirals around the oval.

'Do you still want to?' I ask.

'I don't know,' says Pavan. 'Can we?'

'It kind of sounds like the right amount of stupid. A wedding in a week.'

We look up the rules: weddings are allowed, but only in COVID-safe venues with fewer than twenty people in attendance. Pavan looks at our coffee cups.

'What about Rodney's?' he says.

He means the small cafe-slash-antique shop off St Georges Road. We were getting our coffees there throughout the lockdowns. The coffee isn't the best on the street, but we've grown to like the owner. Somewhere between lockdowns three and four, he became less like a stranger, and more like a friend.

We rush to his store, giddily pitch him the idea.

'You're kidding,' he says. 'I literally just got a delivery of twelve candelabras.'

We take it as a sign, call Julie back.

I keep tracing the threads of this illness around and around, trying to find a neat conclusion. I imagine how this would end in a horror film: the illness conquered, bloody, slain. A moment of relief as the world returns to normal, and then—at the final moment—an eerie movement or shadow, an allusion to the monster's return. In some ways, that is my ending. My mood improves with treatment but imperfectly so. There are still months in which I sink to previous lows. The monster always returns.

I think of Carrie, and how her story ended with death. I think of *Jennifer's Body*, and how Jennifer's friend Needy ended up in an insane asylum. I think of *Raw*, and how Justine learned that this monstrosity was not just hers, but her mother's and sister's, too, embedded in the spirals of their DNA. Her sister ended up in prison. Her father sat her down and told her that there were other ways to live. He unbuttoned his shirt, showed her a constellation of scars, and promised her that she would find a way to cope. I think that I am learning to cope, too.

I've read so many stories of women who were dealt worse hands than mine. Women who were confined, institutionalised, incarcerated, not believed. I found their stories in medical records and case notes, yet no matter how helpful or honest or informative these documents were, I could not find what I was looking for—the direct experience of the illness. I learned what these women had done, but that could not explain for me the fullness of what they felt, or who they were. I thought that I was trying to fill the gaps in my memory, to understand what I was capable of, but perhaps I was just looking for myself on the page, my story written for me, the ending neat and solid and manageable.

While writing this, I searched through my own medical records, too. As in my memory, there are gaps. The portrait I see is a Frankenstein's monster of subjective half-truths sewn together to represent something that is both me and wholly other. In one file, I have a 'child-like affect'; in another, I am a 'pleasant, cooperative and well-engaged woman'. Each of these documents feels too rational and removed to capture the whole of the story. It is easier, I suppose, to believe that a monster tried to kill me than it is to imagine 'sudden intense suicidal ideation that lasted approximately sixteen hours'.

Neither monsters nor medicine alone can tell the whole truth of what happened to me during the worst of this illness, in the worst of the lockdowns. I'm starting to fill in the gaps with the only thing I have: myself, my body, my own experience.

In *Illness as Metaphor*, Susan Sontag pushes back against the metaphors we use to describe illnesses, and the way we use illnesses as metaphors of their own. The narratives we shape around illness, and the stigmas they carry, can bend our experiences of them. I think of werewolves and curses and wandering wombs. I think of thousands of years of narrative and metaphor avalanching over me as I experience my own illness on a cold day in March, spiralling through story after story. Sometimes an illness just is. Sometimes the healthiest way to be ill is to be ill without a story.

On the day of our wedding, a sixth lockdown is announced. We read about it on our phones as we wait to say our vows. It barely comes as a surprise. This feels normal—expected, even. The universe doesn't want us to get married, but now it's too late.

The cafe-slash-antique shop is in an old brick terrace with a shop window out the front and living quarters behind and above. The storefront is filled with mismatched rows of antique chairs and benches. We're waiting in the hallway behind the cafe, on the stairs leading up to the owner's bedroom. On the other side of the wall, I can hear voices, laughter. The wedding has started. We rush through the vows, the photos, the speeches. I have the sudden realisation that I won't see my friends and family for a while. *What a way to say goodbye*, I think.

By 8 p.m., our wedding is over, and we're back in lockdown. Pavan and I walk home, pop the champagne no one had time to drink. We dance in the living room.

'You have to choose to stop somewhere,' writes Carmen Maria Machado in her memoir, *In the Dream House*. If this were a romance novel, perhaps I'd end it here, but life does and did go on. One reality about living with chronic illness is that there is no neat ending, only new moments. In writing about life, about illness, I am choosing to craft a new path between the narratives that helped me, and the narratives that didn't.

It has been ten years since I was first diagnosed with PMDD. I hope and believe this will all be different in another ten years. My endocrinologist believes so, too. Everything moves slowly, and then all at once. Likely within a decade, there will be a new medication that will stop my tidal moods without reducing the rest of me. Perhaps in a similar timeframe our scientific understanding of this illness will grow stronger than centuries of constructed myths. Until then, I am learning to only be monstrous in the ways that I want to be, and to allow multiple stories to be true all at once.

Two days after our wedding, Pavan dropped me at the airport in Tullamarine. He pulled up outside the departures terminal and we hugged until I felt a familiar weepiness coming on. There was no one there to wave us along, or to say we were holding up traffic. I'd never seen the terminal so empty; my flight was the only one on the departures board.

'Well, goodbye,' I said.

'Yup, this is it.'

'See you in three years.'

'Goodbye forever.'

I cry-laughed, squeezed him one more time, then walked away. Over my shoulder, I could see Pavan waiting by the car, waving at me until I was inside the airport. We'd spent a year and a half living on top of one another. I didn't know if we could make long distance work, didn't know if we would work. It didn't feel like an ending, or a beginning, but something new.

Acknowledgements

This book was written on the unceded land of the Wurundjeri people of the Kulin Nation, and the land of the Nuwuvi, or Southern Paiute, people in the Mojave Desert. I am grateful to have been able to live and make art in these very special places.

I want to thank my early readers and mentors in Vegas: Douglas Unger, David Morris, Laura Shaw and Danielle Roth-Johnson. Thank you to Maile Chapman for your psychic-like readings of early drafts. Thank you Arel, for all the mornings spent writing in your living room.

And Amarlie, for having my back both in the Wild (Wild!) West and at home.

To my agent, Michaela McGuire: thank you, thank you, thank you. I'm so glad Hilary pushed me to reach out to you. I couldn't ask for a fiercer advocate. I love that you get both me and my Buffy references. Fate!

Thank you to my publisher, Alex Craig, and the team at Allen & Unwin. I feel endlessly lucky to have found a home with you.

And to my parents. See? It wasn't early childhood trauma. You're off the hook. (Also, Mum: you're taller than you look and great at parallel parking.)

Finally, Pavan. Without you I cannot imagine this book, nor the kinds of stories I might still be telling myself. Thank you for making me laugh. Still looking forward to the divorce party, though it seems less likely by the day.

Works cited

1.

Alison, Jane, *Meander Spiral Explode*, New York: Catapult, 2019

Bolte Taylor, Jill, *My Stroke of Insight: A brain scientist's personal journey*, London: Hodder & Stoughton, 2009

Brugler, Mercer R. et al., 'The transcriptome of the Bermuda fireworm *Odontosyllis enopla* (Annelida: Syllidae): A unique luciferase gene family and putative epitoky-related genes', *PloS ONE*, 2018, vol. 13, no. 8, e0200944, doi:10.1371/journal.pone.0200944

Chu, Jennifer, 'The growth of an organism rides on a pattern of waves', *MIT News*, Massachusetts Institute of Technology, <https://news.mit.edu/2020/growth-organism-waves-0323>, 23 March 2020

Kelleher, Shannon, 'Moon cycles exert an influence on menstruation and sleep patterns', American Association for the Advancement of Science, <www.aaas.org/news/moon-cycles-exert-influence-menstruation-and-sleep-patterns>, 28 January 2021

Kronauer, Daniel J., *Army Ants: Nature's ultimate social hunters*, Cambridge, MA: Harvard University Press, 2020

Markandeya, Virat, 'How lunar cycles guide the spawning of sea creatures', *Smithsonian Magazine*, <www.smithsonianmag.com/science-nature/how-lunar-cycles-guide-the-spawning-of-sea-creatures-180981732>, 8 March 2023

'Spirals in nature: Why this pattern is so common', *Biology Insights*, <biologyinsights.com/spirals-in-nature-why-this-pattern-is-so-common/>, 3 August 2025

3.

Alaimo, Stacy, 'Your shell on acid: Material immersion, Anthropocene dissolves', in *Exposed: Environmental politics and pleasures in posthuman times*, Minneapolis: University of Minnesota Press, 2016, pp. 143–68

4.

Brooks, Jeanne, Diane Ruble and Anne Clark, 'College women's attitudes and expectations concerning menstrual-related changes', *Psychosomatic Medicine*, 1977, vol. 39, no. 5, pp. 288–98, doi:10.1097/00006842-197709000-00002

Bures, Frank, 'Got PMS? Thank our menstruation-fearing culture, not biology', *Slate Magazine*, <https://slate.com/technology/2016/11/pms-might-be-a-cultural-syndrome-not-a-biologic-one.html>, 28 November 2016

Cosgrove, Lisa and Bethany Riddle, 'Constructions of femininity and experiences of menstrual distress', *Women & Health*, 2008, vol. 38, no. 3, pp. 37–58, doi:10.1300/J013v38n03_04

Gurevich, Maria, 'Rethinking the label: Who benefits from the PMS construct?' *Women & Health*, 1995, vol. 23, no. 2, pp. 67–98, doi:10.1300/J013v23n02_05

5.

Boorse, Christopher, 'Premenstrual syndrome and criminal responsibility', in Benson E. Ginsburg and Bonnie Frank Carter (eds), *Premenstrual Syndrome: Ethical and legal implications in a biomedical perspective*, New York: Plenum Press, 1987, pp. 81–124

Bourgault du Coudray, Chantal, 'The cycle of the werewolf: Romantic ecologies of selfhood in popular fantasy', *Australian Feminist Studies*, 2003, vol. 18, no. 40, pp. 57–72, doi:10.1080/0816464022000056376

Briefel, Aviva, 'Monster pains: Masochism, menstruation and identification in the horror film', *Film Quarterly*, 2005, vol. 58, no. 3, pp. 16–27, doi:10.1525/fq.2005.58.3.16

'British courts recognize female "tension" as defence', UPI, <www.upi.com/Archives/1981/11/11/British-courts-recognize-female-tension-as-defense/3478374302800/>, 11 November 1981

'British courts say "yes": Premenstrual tension: Defense for murder?', *Daily Kent Stater*, <https://dks.library.kent.edu/?a=d&d=dks19820218-01.2.52>, 18 February 1982, p. 14

Chambers, Marcia, 'Premenstrual stresses as a legal defense', *The New York Times*, 29 May 1982, p. 46

Cininas, Jazmina, 'Beware the full moon: Female werewolves and "that time of the month"', unpublished paper, supplied to the author December 2023

Cohen, Jeffrey Jerome (ed), *Monster Theory: Reading culture*, Minneapolis: University of Minnesota Press, 1996

McSherry, Bernadette, 'The return of the raging hormones theory', *Sydney Law Review*, 1993, vol. 15, no. 3, pp. 292–316

Notre Dame Law Review Editors, 'Recent decisions', *Notre Dame Law Review*, 1983, vol. 59, no. 1, <https://scholarship.law.nd.edu/ndlr/vol59/iss1/11>

'Once in a Blue Moon', *Charmed*, season 7, episode 6, created by Constance M. Burge, The WB, 2004

Solomon, Lee, 'Premenstrual syndrome: The debate surrounding criminal defense', *Maryland Law Review*, 1995, vol. 54, no. 2, pp. 571–600, <http://digitalcommons.law.umaryland.edu/mlr/vol54/iss2/10>

Thakur, C. P. and Dilip Sharma, 'Full moon and crime', *British Medical Journal*, 1984, vol. 289, pp. 1789–91, doi:10.1136/bmj.289.6460.1789

The Curse, directed by Jacqueline Garry, Arrow Entertainment, 1999

The Howling, directed by Joe Dante, Embassy Pictures, 1981

6.

Garner, Helen, interview by Erik Jensen, 'Hotel Golf', *The Monthly*, <www.themonthly.com.au/june-2018/essays/hotel-golf>, June 2018

Serpell, James and Priscilla Barrett, *The Domestic Dog: Its evolution, behavior and interactions with people*, 2nd edn, Cambridge: Cambridge University Press, 2017

8.

Breuer, Josef and Sigmund Freud, *Studies on Hysteria*, translated by James Strachey, New York: Basic Books, 1957

Cininas, 'Beware the full moon'

Cohut, Maria, 'The controversy of "female hysteria"', *Medical News Today*, <www.medicalnewstoday.com/articles/the-controversy-of-female-hysteria>, 13 October 2020

Freud, Sigmund, 'Hysteria', in James Strachey and Anna Freud (eds), *The Standard Edition of the Complete Psychological Works of Sigmund Freud, Volume I (1886–1899): Pre-psycho-analytic publications and unpublished drafts*, New York: Vintage, 1966, pp. 37–59

——'Letter from Freud to Fliess, September 21, 1897', in Jeffrey Masson (ed), *The Complete Letters of Sigmund Freud to Wilhelm Fliess, 1887–1904*, Psychoanalytic Electronic Publishing, pp. 264–7, <https://pep-web.org/search/document/ZBK.042.0264A?page=P0264>

Gilman, Charlotte Perkins, *The Yellow Wallpaper*, London: Virago Press, 1981

——'Why I wrote "The Yellow Wallpaper"', in Arielle Zibrak (ed), *Twelve Stories by American Women*, New York: Penguin Classics, 2025, via *Literary Hub*, <https://lithub.com/charlotte-perkins-gilman-on-why-she-wrote-the-yellow-wallpaper/>, 19 March 2025

Goetz, Christopher G., 'Jean-Martin Charcot and Silas Weir Mitchell', *Neurology*, 1997, vol. 48, no. 4, pp. 1128–32, doi:10.1212/wnl.48.4.1128

Greene, Raymond and Katharina Dalton, 'The premenstrual syndrome', *British Medical Journal*, 1953, vol. 1, no. 4818, pp. 1007–14, doi:10.1136/bmj.1.4818.1007

Sarmiento, Sofia, 'The lingering effects of female hysteria in medicine', *Berkeley Political Review*, <https://bpr.berkeley.edu/2021/08/10/the-lingering-effects-of-female-hysteria-in-medicine/>, 10 August 2021

Waraich, Manni and Shailesh Shah, 'The life and work of Jean-Martin Charcot (1825–1893): "The Napoleon of Neuroses"', *Journal of the Intensive Care Society*, 2018, vol. 19, no. 1, pp. 48–9, doi:10.1177/1751143717709420

Woolf, Virginia, *Mrs Dalloway*, London: Vintage, 2004

9.

Carrie, directed by Brian De Palma, United Artists, 1976

Cininas, Jazmina, 'Wicked wolf-women and shaggy suffragettes: Lycanthropic femmes fatales in the Victorian and Edwardian eras', in Robert McKay and John Miller (eds), *Werewolves, Wolves and the Gothic*, Cardiff: University of Wales Press, 2017, pp. 37–64

Cixous, Hélène, 'The laugh of the Medusa', translated by Keith Cohen and Paula Cohen, in Vincent B. Leitch (ed), *The Norton Anthology of Theory and Criticism*, 1st edn, New York: W.W. Norton & Company, 2001, pp. 2039–56

Cohen, *Monster Theory*

King, Stephen, *Carrie*, London: Hodder & Stoughton, 2004

Psycho, directed by Alfred Hitchcock, Paramount Pictures, 1960

Whiteley, Kathleen, 'Hippocrates' *Diseases of Women Book I*: Greek text with English translation and footnotes', University of South Africa, Pretoria, 2009, <http://hdl.handle.net/10500/1620>

Zimmerman, Jess, *Women and Other Monsters: Building a new mythology*, Boston, MA: Beacon Press, 2021

11.

Battlestar Galactica: The miniseries, created by Ronald D. Moore and David Eick, Universal Television LLC, 2003

Butler, Kirstin, 'Life-saving tool or torture device?', *American Experience*, PBS, <https://pbs.org/wgbh/americanexperience/features/cancer-detectives-brief-history-speculum/>, 15 March 2024

Carrie, directed by De Palma

Cohen, *Monster Theory*

Haraway, Donna J., 'A manifesto for cyborgs: Science, technology and socialist feminism in the 1980s', in Vincent B. Leitch (ed), *The Norton Anthology of Theory and Criticism*, 1st edn, New York: W.W. Norton & Company, 2001, pp. 2269–99

Shelley, Mary, *Frankenstein*, London: Vintage, 2019

Vatanoğlu-Lutz, E. Elif and Ahmet Doğan Ataman, 'Medicine in philately: Rene T. H. Laënnec, the father of stethoscope', *Anatolian Journal of Cardiology*, 2016, vol. 16, no. 2, pp. 146–7, doi:10.14744/AnatolJCardiol.2015.6866

Zimmerman, *Women and Other Monsters*

12.

American Psychiatric Association, 'Premenstrual syndrome', in *Diagnostic and Statistical Manual of Mental Disorders, Fifth Edition, (DSM-V)*, American Psychiatric Association Publishing, 2013

'Bipolar disorder and PMDD', iapmd.org, <https://iapmd.org/pmdd-bipolar-disorder>, 4 November 2020

Boorse, 'Premenstrual syndrome and criminal responsibility'

Breuer and Freud, *Studies on Hysteria*

'British courts recognize female "tension" as defence', UPI

'British courts say "yes"', *Daily Kent Stater*

Chrisler, Joan C., 'Hormone hostages: The cultural legacy of PMS as a legal defense', in Lynn H. Collins, Michelle R. Dunlap and Joan C. Chrisler (eds), *Charting a New Course for Feminist Psychology*, Westport: Praeger Publishers, 2002, pp. 238–52

Endicott, Jean, 'History, evolution, and diagnosis of premenstrual dysphoric disorder', *The Journal of Clinical Psychiatry*, 2000, vol. 61, suppl. 12, pp. 5–8

Frank, Robert T., 'The hormonal causes of premenstrual tension', *Archives of Neurology and Psychiatry*, 1931, vol. 26, no. 5, pp. 1053–7, doi:10.1001/archneurpsyc.1931.02230110151009

Freud, 'Hysteria'

Holtzman, Elizabeth, 'Premenstrual syndrome: No legal defense', letter to the editor, *St. John's Law Review*, 1986, vol. 60, no. 4, pp. 712–15

Houppert, Karen, *The Curse: Confronting the last unmentionable taboo: Menstruation*, New York: Farrar, Straus and Giroux, 1999

Kieckhefer, Richard, *European Witch Trials: Their foundations in popular and learned culture, 1300–1500*, Berkeley and Los Angeles: University of California Press, 1976

King, Sally, 'Premenstrual syndrome (PMS) and the myth of the irrational female', in Chris Bobel et al. (eds), *The Palgrave Handbook of Critical Menstruation Studies*, Singapore: Palgrave Macmillan, 2020, pp. 287–302

Machado, Carmen Maria, *In the Dream House*, Minneapolis: Graywolf Press, 2019

McSherry, Bernadette, 'Premenstrual syndrome and criminal responsibility', *Psychiatry, Psychology and Law*, 1994, vol. 1, no. 2, pp. 131–51, doi:10.1080/13218719409524837

——'The return of the raging hormones theory'

Micale, Mark S., 'On the "disappearance" of hysteria: A study in the clinical deconstruction of a diagnosis', *Isis*, 1993, vol. 84, no. 3, pp. 496–526, <www.jstor.org/stable/235644>

Notre Dame Law Review Editors, 'Recent decisions'

Ro, Christine, 'The overlooked condition that can trigger extreme behaviour', BBC, <www.bbc.com/future/article/20191213-pmdd-a-little-understood-and-often-misdiagnosed-condition>, 16 December 2019

Solomon, 'Premenstrual syndrome'

Studd, John, 'Severe premenstrual syndrome and bipolar disorder: A tragic confusion', *Menopause International*, 2012, vol. 18, no. 2, pp. 82–6, doi:10.1258/mi.2012.012018

Zachary, Peter and Kenneth S. Kendler, 'Section 14: The decision to include or exclude a diagnosis in psychiatric nosology: The case of premenstrual dysphoric disorder', in Kenneth S. Kendler and Josef Parnas (eds), *Philosophical Issues in Psychology III*, Oxford: Oxford University Press, 2014, pp. 349-71

Zimmerman, *Women and Other Monsters*

13.

Houppert, *The Curse*

Tolentino, Jia, *Trick Mirror: Reflections on self-delusion*, London: HarperCollins, 2019

14.

Sontag, Susan, *Illness as Metaphor*, New York: Farrar, Straus and Giroux, 1978

Qadar, Sana, '"Like a bereavement every month"—the extreme emotions of PMDD', *All in the Mind*, ABC, <www.abc.net.au/listen/programs/allinthemind/extreme-emotions-pmdd-premenstrual-dysphoric-disorder/102373574>, 4 June 2023

15.

Stevenson, Robert Louis, *The Strange Case of Dr Jekyll and Mr Hyde*, London: New English Library, 1974

16.

Baker, David and Natacha Keramidas, 'The psychology of hunger', *Monitor on Psychology*, 2013, vol. 44, no. 9, <www.apa.org/monitor/2013/10/hunger>

Harkins-Cross, Rebecca, 'Only women bleed', *The Lifted Brow*, 2017, vol. 34, pp. 5–8

Henery, Molly, '*Jennifer's Body* and other teenage hells', *Certified Forgotten*, <https://certifiedforgotten.com/jennifers-body/>, 27 April 2021

Jennifer's Body, directed by Karyn Kusama, 20th Century Fox, 2009

Kang, Han, *The Vegetarian*, translated by Deborah Smith, London: Portobello Books, 2015

Raw, directed by Julia Ducournau, Wild Bunch, 2016

Teeth, directed by Mitchell Lichtenstein, Pierpoline Films, 2007

University of California, Berkeley, 'Lack of females in drug dose trials leads to overmedicated women', *ScienceDaily*, <www.sciencedaily.com/releases/2020/08/200812161318.htm>, 12 August 2020

17.

Foucault, Michel, *The Birth of the Clinic: An archaeology of medical perception*, translated by Alan Sheridan, London: Tavistock, 1973

18.

Gibson, Megan, 'The long strange history of birth control', *Time Magazine*, <https://time.com/3692001/birth-control-history-djerassi/>, 3 February 2015

Jackson, Jhoni, 'How Puerto Rican women made birth control possible—at the expense of their health', *BESE*, <https://web.archive.org/

web/20230330062306/https://www.bese.com/how-puerto-rican-women-made-birth-control-possible-at-the-expense-of-their-health/>, 2018

'Male birth control study killed after men report side effects', *All Things Considered*, NPR, <www.npr.org/sections/health-shots/2016/11/03/500549503/male-birth-control-study-killed-after-men-complain-about-side-effects>, 3 November 2016

May, Elaine Tyler, *America and the Pill: A history of promise, peril, and liberation*, 1st edn, New York: Basic Books, 2010

Pendergrass, Drew C. and Michelle Y. Raji, 'The bitter pill: Harvard and the dark history of birth control', *The Crimson*, <www.thecrimson.com/article/2017/9/28/the-bitter-pill/>, 28 September 2017

Roberts, William C., 'Facts and ideas from anywhere: "The pill" and its four major developers', *Baylor University Medical Center Proceedings*, 2015, vol. 28, no. 3, pp. 421–32, doi:10.1080/08998280.2015.11929297

'Roots of the pill', *American Experience*, PBS, <www.pbs.org/wgbh/americanexperience/features/roots-pill/>, accessed 17 August 2025

Ryan, Lisa, 'No, the male birth control study wasn't halted because men couldn't handle the side-effects', *The Cut*, <www.thecut.com/2016/11/the-real-reason-the-male-birth-control-study-was-halted.html>, 3 November 2016

Sanger, Margaret, *The Pivot of Civilization*, Project Gutenberg, <https://www.gutenberg.org/cache/epub/1689/pg1689-images.html#link2HCH0001>, 22 February 2006

Weber, Max, *The Protestant Ethic and the Spirit of Capitalism*, translated by Talcott Parsons, London: Routledge, 2001

20.

Bryant, Katerina, *Hysteria: A memoir of illness, strength and women's stories throughout history*, Sydney: NewSouth, 2020

Nietzsche, Friedrich, 'On truth and lies in a non-moral sense', in Vincent B. Leitch (ed), *The Norton Anthology of Theory and Criticism*, 1st edn, New York: W.W. Norton & Company, 2001, pp. 870–4

21.

Chen, Shiyi et al., 'Allopregnanolone in mood disorders: Mechanism and therapeutic development', *Pharmacological Research*, 2021, vol. 169, 105682, doi:10.1016/j.phrs.2021.105682

22.

Chen et al., 'Allopregnanolone in mood disorders'

Darbra, Sònia and Marc Pallarès, 'Developmental actions of neurosteroids in rodents: Focus on allopregnanolone', *Current Opinion in Endocrine and Metabolic Research*, 2022, vol. 23, 100317, doi:10.1016/j.coemr.2022.100317

Raw, directed by Ducournau

Wei, Sheng et al., 'A forced swim-based rat model of premenstrual depression: Effects of hormonal changes and drug intervention', *Aging*, 2020, vol. 12, no. 23, pp. 24357–70, doi:10.18632/aging.202249

23.

'Dialectic Behavioral Therapy Program', Hartford HealthCare Institute of Living, <https://instituteofliving.org/programs-services/adult-services/departments-services/dialectic-behavioral-therapy-program>, accessed 17 August 2025

Linehan, Marsha M. and Chelsey R. Wilks, 'The course and evolution of Dialectical Behavior Therapy', *American Journal of Psychotherapy*, 2015, vol. 69, no. 2, pp. 97–110, doi:10.1176/appi.psychotherapy.2015.69.2.97

Linehan, Marsha M., 'Dialectical Behavior Therapy for treatment of borderline personality disorder: Implications for the treatment of substance abuse', *NIDA Research Monograph*, 1993, vol. 137, pp. 201–16, PMID:8289922

'Mont Park Hospital', Victorian Government, <https://www.vic.gov.au/mont-park-hospital>, 17 June 2025

Reid, Laurie, 'History of psychiatric care', Mont Park to Springthorpe, <https://www.montparktospringthorpe.com/history-of-psychiatric-care/>, 7 May 2018

25.

Australian Human Rights Commission, *Older Women's Risk of Homelessness: Background paper*, <https://humanrights.gov.au/our-work/age-discrimination/publications/older-womens-risk-homelessness-background-paper-2019>, April 2019

Delaney, Janice, Mary Jane Lupton and Emily Toth, *The Curse: A cultural history of menstruation*, New York: Dutton, 1976

Hantsoo, Liisa and C. Neill Epperson, 'Allopregnanolone in premenstrual dysphoric disorder (PMDD): Evidence for dysregulated sensitivity to GABA-A receptor modulating neuroactive steroids across the menstrual cycle', *Neurobiology of Stress*, 2020, vol. 12, 100213, doi:10.1016/j.ynstr.2020.100213

——'Premenstrual dysphoric disorder: Epidemiology and treatment', *Current Psychiatry Reports*, 2015, vol. 17, no. 11, article 87, doi:10.1007/s11920-015-0628-3

Houppert, *The Curse*

LeWine, Howard E., 'The power of the placebo effect', *Harvard Health*, <https://www.health.harvard.edu/mental-health/the-power-of-the-placebo-effect>, 22 July 2024

Mukherjee, Siddhartha, 'Post-Prozac nation', *The New York Times*, <www.nytimes.com/2012/04/22/magazine/the-science-and-history-of-treating-depression.html>, 19 April 2012

National Center for Biotechnology Information, 'PubChem compound summary for CID 3386, Fluoxetine', *PubChem*, <https://pubchem.ncbi.nlm.nih.gov/compound/Fluoxetine>, accessed 20 February 2024

Offill, Jenny, *Dept. of Speculation*, London: Granta, 2014

Raw, directed by Ducournau

26.

Martinez, Pedro E. et al, '5α-Reductase inhibition prevents the luteal phase increase in plasma allopregnanolone levels and mitigates symptoms in women with premenstrual dysphoric disorder', *Neuropsychopharmacol.* 2015, vol. 41, pp. 1093–102, doi:10.1038/npp.2015.246

27.

van der Kolk, Bessel, *The Body Keeps the Score*, New York: Penguin Publishing Group, 2014

28.

Benjamin, Marlene, 'The disordered self: Philosophy, memoir and madness', in Gonzalo Araoz, Fátima Alves and Katrina Jaworski (eds), *Rethinking Madness: Interdisciplinary and multicultural reflections*, Leiden, the Netherlands: Brill, 2013, pp. 27–50

29.

Carrie, directed by De Palma
Jennifer's Body, directed by Kusama
Machado, *In the Dream House*
Raw, directed by Ducournau
Smith, Ali, 'True short story', *European Journal of English Studies*, 2006, vol. 10, no. 3, pp. 283–7, doi:10.1080/13825570600967747
Sontag, *Illness as Metaphor*